Challenges of Interpreting
Between Hmong Patients
& Western Medicine

Challenges of Interpreting Between Hmong Patients & Western Medicine

An Interpreter's Perspective

Maiv Txiab Vam Xeeb Yaj

Copyright © 2014 by Maiv Txiab Vam Xeeb Yaj.

Library of Congress Control Number: 2014920010
ISBN: Hardcover   978-1-4990-8073-5
         Softcover   978-1-4990-8075-9
         eBook   978-1-4990-8074-2

All rights reserved. No part of this book may be reproduced or transmitted in any form or by any means, electronic or mechanical, including photocopying, recording, or by any information storage and retrieval system, without permission in writing from the copyright owner.

Any people depicted in stock imagery provided by Dreamstime are models, and such images are being used for illustrative purposes only. Certain stock imagery © Dreamstime.

Cover design by "Yang Design www.yangdesign.net"

This book was printed in the United States of America.

Rev. date: 12/15/2014

To order additional copies of this book, contact:
Xlibris
1-888-795-4274
www.Xlibris.com
Orders@Xlibris.com
695887

CONTENTS

Acknowledgments 7
Introduction 9

Chapter One: My Observations of Culture
               Misinterpretation 13

   Case No. 1:   Broken Bones 16
   Case No. 2:   Private Areas 21
   Case No. 3:   Killer Pills 25
   Case No. 4:   Burning Bananas 29
   Case No. 5:   The Traumatic Ear 35
   Case No. 6:   Silent Birth 39
   Case No. 7:   Hospital Sleepover 45
   Case No. 8:   Water Medicine 48
   Case No. 9:   Interpreter Becomes the Patient 52
   Case No. 10: Death and Dying 57

Chapter Two: Effective Utilization of an Interpreter by
               American Medical Providers 69

   Case No. 1:   Turn-Taking Method
                 (Consecutive Interpreting) 70
   Case No. 2:   All-at-Once Method (Difficulty of
                 Simultaneous Interpreting by Phone) 73
   Case No. 3:   Speak Slowly and Clearly Method
                 (Consecutive Interpreting/Asking for
                 Clarifications as Needed) 76

Case No. 4: Talk-to-the-Appropriate-Person Method (Know How and Whom to Ask for the Information You Seek) 80

Chapter Three: Closing Thoughts on the Challenges of Interpreting Different Worldviews 86

Epilogue 92

Acknowledgments

I would like to take this opportunity to thank the medical doctors, nurses, social workers, and other professional staffs who work with our elderly and new immigrant Hmong patients, who also do not speak English. Despite the frustrations and misunderstandings that come with not speaking the same language, you try your best to help our sick non–English speaking Hmong patients get better. I also would like to thank those of you who supported me and those of you who have taken the time to read my book—to not only understand what I go through every day, but also to deepen your understanding about the real challenges of interpreting between different cultures.

I would like to thank my supportive husband, Paul Moua, who graduated from Metropolitan Community College in Omaha, Nebraska, with an Associate Degree in Electronics. Paul continued his education and graduated from California State University, Stanislaus, California, with a Bachelor's Degree in Business Administration. He also graduated from National University in Sacramento, California, with a Master's Degree in Business Administration. Paul has been working for Valley Mountain Regional Center in Modesto, California, for seventeen years. I also acknowledge my three children—Christie, Charlie, and Valerie—who were always there to help me whenever I needed them. I would also like to thank my sweet mother, Mrs. Wa Seng Yang; my older sister, Mai Youa Yang; and my brother-in-law Peter Chang. They have all helped me in explaining and sharing our Hmong culture, history, and spiritual beliefs in this book.

Last but not least are the two most important people in my life that I would like to thank. One of them is my younger brother, Lee Yang, who attended the University of Wisconsin–Madison for his undergraduate degree, and who has been working as a professional and CoreCHI Certified Medical and Legal Interpreter in Madison, Wisconsin, for the past twenty years. And the second person is my younger sister, Nou Yang, who has helped me with the initial thought process of putting this book together, bounced and refined ideas, and did the draft proofreads and revisions. She also attended and received her Master's Degree from the University of Wisconsin–Madison for Bicultural Competency of Hmong Teens, and now she is currently working as the Director of the Youth Leadership Initiative at Wilder Foundation, and is a board member of Hnub Tshiab: Hmong Women Achieving Together in St. Paul, Minnesota. Both my younger brother, Lee, and sister, Nou Yang, helped me review and edit my book several times. Brother and Sister, without you two, I would not be able to make my dream come true. Again, thank you both for your love and significant support.

Introduction

I have been interpreting for more than twenty years at a medical clinic, mental health clinic, and over-the-phone interpreting services. After graduating from community college, I worked as a receptionist, cashier, data-entry clerk, billing clerk, assistant supervisor, and interpreted at a health clinic for many Hmong patients in the past who did not know much English when they came to see their primary physicians and other medical staffs. While I was working at the health clinic, I also worked as a part-time Hmong interpreter for a mental health clinic with many Hmong clients who had been affected with post-traumatic stress disorder (PTSD) from the Vietnam War. At the present time, I am working as an over-the-phone Hmong interpreter for a company and other previous companies, interpreting for hospitals, doctors' offices, mental health clinics, welfare departments, police stations, medical billing, phone bills, utility bills, life insurance, Internet issues, airports, jails, nursing homes, hospices, dental offices, and others.

Based on my work experiences, I would consider the phone interpretation services as the most challenging, because over the phone I can only use my imagination to communicate with the doctors, nurses, and non–English-speaking Hmong patients; and I cannot use any of my facial expressions, hand gestures, or body language to help clarify misunderstandings. Since I have been working as a Hmong interpreter for a long time, I have noticed and realized that being the middle person is a very difficult task, especially in interpreting over the phone and you can't see people. I hope that this book will help shed light on the challenges of phone interpretation and help bridge the cultural misunderstandings between professional medical staffs and non–English-speaking Hmong patients or clients.

There are many other reasons why it is difficult working as an interpreter. I have found that the older Hmong generations who grew up in Laos and came to the United States after the Vietnam War in 1975 are the most difficult to translate and interpret for, because their worldview is so different from the Western worldview. Every time I interpret between the Western and the Hmong culture, I notice this cultural difference. In Western culture, when we speak, we like to speak very direct and to the point so we can finish the conversation faster; but for the Hmong culture, we like to speak very indirectly because it is viewed as being disrespectful and rude to say directly what you want. For Hmong people, if we speak indirectly, it is because we respect the other person and do not want to show off that we are better than the other person. That is why the majority of our older Hmong patients may seem to beat around the bush a lot rather than speak very directly.

As the interpreter, I am expected to quickly interpret to the best of my knowledge for both Western and Hmong cultures within minutes. For example, if the word is *daj ntseg* in the Hmong language and you did a literal interpreting and/or translation, it would mean "yellow ear." The correct interpretation or translation in meaning is "jaundice" or "pale." As someone who has an insider's cultural knowledge and understanding of both worldviews, I feel the responsibility to also assist in cultural interpretation, while managing cultural nuisances on topics such as death and dying and other sensitive topics. This slows down the process significantly, and oftentimes, I have to be the one to ask the Western medical personnel to pause from talking in order to explain how culture is impacting the conversation or what the non–English-speaking Hmong patient understands of the medical instruction or the doctor's questions.

I hope that my experiences and this book will help (1) both cultures to better understand the other's perspectives, (2) the medical field to provide more culturally sensitive health-care services to non–English-speaking Hmong patients, particularly the elderly, and (3) to recognize that as the middle person, interpreters or translators are not just providing language interpretation or translation but also cultural interpretation, which is the key to successful communication and understanding between a non–English-speaking patient and a Western or English speaking medical staff. Having cultural knowledge and the ability to appropriately interpret are very important.

The intent of my book is not to go into great depth about the theory, modes and best practices of language interpretation, but merely to share my own personal experiences about the difficulties of language and cultural misunderstandings and assumptions; particularly when working with older non–English-speaking Hmong patients.

Prior to coming to the United States, most of older Hmong people never received any formal education; many do not even know how to read and write their own language. Once in the United States, although the literacy rate improved due to access to education, many older Hmong people struggled to learn the English language and continued to rely on their children or grandchildren who grew up or were born in the United States to assist them with language interpretation and translation.

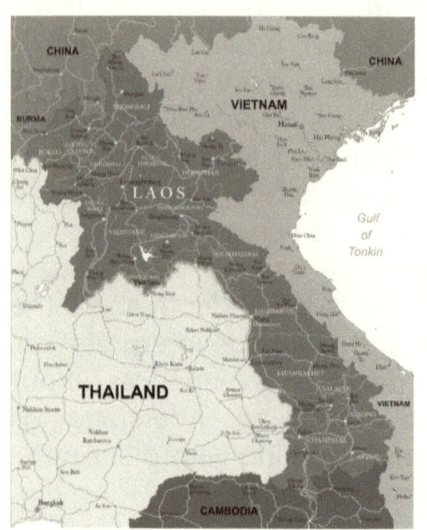

Map of Laos

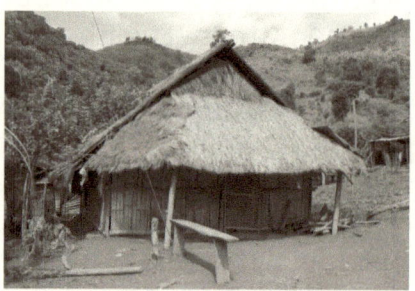

Hmong thatched-housing in Laos.

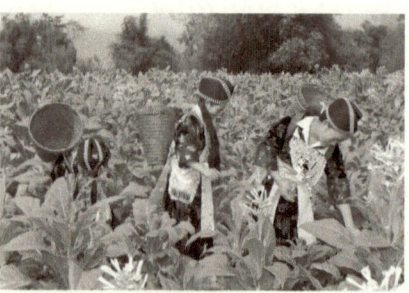

Hmong people working at the farm in Laos.

Chapter One

My Observations of Culture Misinterpretation

I know that my job is to interpret from one language to the other, word for word without losing the critical meaning. But sometimes it did not happen that way at all. Because the older and new immigrant Hmong patients lack education, it is very difficult to just literally interpret what the American medical staff says. When interpreting word for word to the Hmong patients, the words, sentences, or thoughts did not make any sense to the Hmong patients at all. For example, the word "smart" means that a person is intelligent in the American language. However, in our Hmong language, there are two different meanings: "Smart" can mean intelligent, but "smart" can also be used to describe when a child's bottom has a rash (as interpreted in the Hmong words *ntse* or *pob tw ntse*). For example, you can't say the baby has a smart butt. As the interpreter, I have to use my cultural understanding of the Hmong language and context to correctly explain what the doctor is talking about. I cannot interpret that the child's bottom is smart because it does not make any sense. We all know that a child's bottom does not talk, so I cannot interpret that the child's bottom is smart. When I interpret about the child's rash on his/her bottom, I have to interpret carefully to the parents to make sure they understand their child's bottom has a rash and not that it is smart.

Most of the time, I am unable to interpret directly, word for word, and be straight to the point. I feel that as an interpreter, it is my job to ensure that both the patient and the doctor have a clear understanding of what the other is saying. That is why I feel like I have no choice but to do some cultural explaining of the phrases, thoughts, and cultural nuisances between the American doctors and the older Hmong patients in order for all of us to be on the same page. For example, on average, it would take a Hmong patient about three to five minutes to explain what is happening with him/her to the doctor. The length of the time for me to interpret it would be double that time. Another factor for this doubling in length of time is that our older Hmong patients are very indirect communicators. They like to tell a story about what is happening to them rather than going straight to the health issue that they are dealing with at the present time.

As a Hmong interpreter for many years, I would like to share my experiences and perspective. I hope that this will help American doctors, nurses, and other professional staffs to better understand the communication style of older Hmong patients. Based on their culture and upbringing, the older Hmong patients believe that communicating directly to the point means that either they are disrespecting whomever they are communicating with or implying they know more than the other person. This perspective is in direct contrary to the Western way of thinking. Furthermore, this generation tends to communicate in a circular manner. Rather than focus on the issue at hand, it is important to communicate the origin of the issue—understanding the past is the only way to truly understand the present. This is why older Hmong patients share their whole life stories when you ask them a simple question. They do this because they feel that this is necessary for the doctor to understand exactly why he or she is in the present health condition that he or she is in. Patients would explain to me that when they go to see their primary physicians, they want their doctors to feel comfortable, respected, and connected to them by sharing their past experiences to the present. This would help their doctors understand them better and provide the necessary care that they need.

Being the middle person is the most difficult when it is the older Hmong patients' turn to talk to the American doctors. The patients are typically so often afraid that their doctors will not understand them; therefore, they always want to tell the whole story of their lives to their doctors. They feel that if they did not tell the whole story to their doctors, their doctors would not understand what they have been through and, therefore, may prescribe the wrong medications for them.

In today's world, we live in very diverse communities. Learning how to communicate across cultures requires a great deal of patience, understanding, and willingness to adapt to each other. It is not only in the professional world of interpreting and translation, but many of us also had to deal with providing translation and/or interpretation for family members. I would like to share some of these difficult interpreting cases between non-English speaking Hmong patients and American doctors, nurses, and other professional staffs, so as to highlight how we can better improve the health-care system for everyone. Below, I will share my most complicated phone cases in order for us to learn from the situation and hopefully minimize future cross-cultural miscommunications and misunderstandings. Names have been changed to protect the confidentiality of individuals.

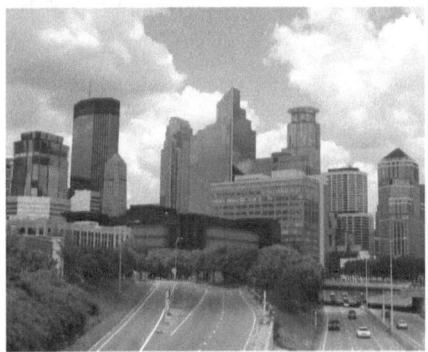

St. Paul, Minnesota. The majority of the Hmong people in the US live in Minnesota, Wisconsin, and California.

Case No. 1: Broken Bones

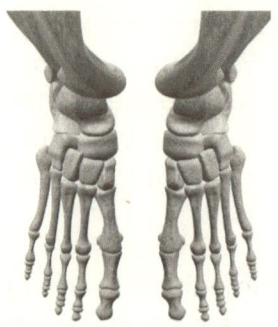

Patient: Hnub Ci Dawb (sixty-five-year-old female patient)

Interpreter: Niam Nkauj Zuag Paj

Location: ER with Dr. Johnson

(Phone Ringing)

Interpreter: Hi, my name is Niam Nkauj Zuag Paj, and my ID number is 11211. I speak Hmong. When you are ready, please go ahead.

Doctor: Hi, I am Dr. Johnson at the hospital. Right now, I am walking into one of the exam rooms. Okay, I am in the room now with the patient. What brings the patient to the ER?

Interpreter: (Interpreted exactly what the doctor said to the patient.)

Patient: I don't know why my right elbow is hurting a lot recently. It has been hurting me for more than two weeks already. Before it only hurt little bit, but now it is hurting me more than ever. It hurts more at night, and I could not sleep at all. I took some Advil for the pain, but it only helped me just for a couple of hours, then the pain came back. Sometimes the pain traveled heavily to my shoulder, my back, my neck, and went up to my head. Especially when my elbow is hurting, I could not touch it or bend it down for a long time. Sometimes I wanted to use my right hand to wash my face, but it hurt so much; so I could not use it at all. Some nights, I felt like cutting it off because it hurt me so much. At nighttime, it seemed like my headache is hurting more. When my headache and my whole body got very bad at night, some nights I ended up having some light fevers, feeling throw up, and also feeling dizziness too.

Interpreter: (Interpreted exactly what the patient just said to the doctor.)

Doctor: Did you fall?

Interpreter: (Interpreted exactly what the doctor said to the patient.)

Patient: No, I did not fall. I am a disabled person. I sit in my wheelchair all day long. I cannot get up, cook, take a shower, and walk around the house, so I did not fall. The person who is helping me around the house is al ways inside the house with me, so I did not have to do anything. When I want to go to the store, she pushes my wheelchair to her car, helps me to get into her car, and she drives me to the store. When we get there, she also helps me to get out of her car; and she helps me to sit on the store handicap automatic shopping car, then I drive the car inside the store to get what I want from the shelves. After I get all my groceries, I drive the store handicap automatic shopping car to the cashier to ring everything and pay. Then my helper (Personal Care Attendant) follows me to her car and puts all the groceries into her car's truck, so we come home. How can I fall?

Interpreter: (Interpreted exactly what the patient said to the doctor.)

Doctor: Any other questions, or any other problems?

Interpreter: (Interpreted exactly what the doctor said to the patient.)

Patient: I would like the doctor to please give me some good medications to take home for my pain because I cannot stand this pain anymore. Sometimes I cannot even touch my elbow at all because it hurts so badly. Since the pain was so painful in the last two weeks and today, I only took a shower twice in the last two weeks. Please give me some good medications so I can feel better and can take a shower sooner. Please tell the doctor that I do not want any surgery. I do not believe that surgery will do any good for me. I think that surgery will do more harm for my elbow, so I rather want to take good medications instead. I believe that for old people like me, maybe the doctors just want to practice on me to have the surgery done only, so I am telling the doctor now that I refuse to have surgery. Old people like me having surgery will take forever to heal back, so I do not want to go through surgery.

Interpreter: (Interpreted exactly what the patient said to the doctor.)

Doctor: If your pain is not going away soon, maybe you need to consider having an X-ray done to see what is wrong inside the bone.

Interpreter: (Interpreted exactly what the doctor said to the patient.)

Patient: No, I do not want any X-ray at all because many years ago, I had a very painful problem on my left leg, and the doctor told me to have the X-ray done, so then I went. But at the end, they did not find anything wrong with my leg, so I think that having the X-ray is just wasting time. Like I said earlier, I did not fall; so my bone is not broken. There is no reason for me to have the X-ray done because I was very scared of the big machine last time. I hope that the doctor understands me and does not force me to have an X-ray done. He is a doctor, so he should understand what I had been through in the past. Please tell the doctor that I did not fall; so that means that the bone did not break.

Interpreter: (Interpreted exactly what the patient said to the doctor.)

Doctor: I will write you a prescription today, so you need to take this prescription to the pharmacy to get the medications for your elbow, okay?

Interpreter: (Interpreted exactly what the doctor said to the patient.)

Doctor: You need to follow up with your primary physician within a week.

Interpreter: (Interpreted exactly what the doctor said to the patient.)

Patient: Okay, thank you.

Interpreter: (Interpreted exactly what the patient said to the doctor.)

Analysis for Case No. 1: Broken Bones

This is a very difficult situation for both parties because of the different cultures. The older Hmong female patient did not understand how the medical process worked exactly. Maybe she thought she just went to talk to the doctor to see if he/she would prescribe some pain medications for her to take only. However, after the doctor listened to her complaints and the pain that she had, the doctor wanted to order her to have the X-ray done because the doctor wanted to see the inside of her arm to make sure nothing was broken.

But for the Hmong patient, she did not understand the doctor's point of view and thought that the pain should disappear after she finished the medication. In her mind, it seemed like she just came for the medications only and nothing else. The moment the doctor was done mentioning about the X-ray, she got very upset and disagreed with the doctor's suggestions right away about the X-ray because she did not experience a recent fall, which would require an X-ray. From the doctor's point of view, he was trying to do everything to help her solve the problem. But the moment the patient heard what the doctor said about the X-ray, she refused it right away because she felt that the X-ray was not necessary. Moreover, surgery was not part of her plan.

Case No. 2: Private Areas

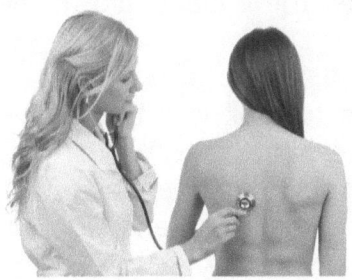

Patient: Mi Nkauj Nog (sixty-seven-year-old female patient who just arrived in America a couple of years ago)

Interpreter: Niam Nkauj Zuag Paj

Nurse: Katy

Location: Regular office visit with Dr. Anderson

(Phone ringing)

Interpreter: Hi, my name is Niam Nkauj Zuag Paj. My ID number is 11211. I speak Hmong. When you are ready, please go head.

Nurse: Hi, my name is Katy. I am a nurse at Dr. Anderson's office. We have a patient in one of the exam rooms for her physical exam. It seems like the patient does not speak English very well. Can you please ask the patient to see if she wants to have general physical and Pap smear today?

Interpreter: (Interpreted exactly what the nurse said to the patient.)

Patient: What is a Pap smear?

Interpreter: (Interpreted exactly what the patient said to the nurse.)

Nurse: A Pap smear is a procedure to look into the female vagina to check to make sure there is no cancer. What the doctor will do is to use a small plastic device to open the cervix, use a quick tip to get some fluids from the inside, and examine the fluids to make sure there is no cancer.

Interpreter: (Interpreted exactly what the nurse said to the patient.)

Patient: I am a very healthy person. If I have any cancer inside of me now, I should start having some kind of pains, right? If I have it, I am pretty sure the cancer would cause a lot of pain inside of me by now, but I am still coming here. No problem then. I do not believe I have cancer. If I ever have the pain, I will call my doctor's office right away, and I will come to see him. I refuse to have my vagina checked today. For today, I am here to have just the general physical only. I do not want the nurse or doctor to see my private area. In Laos—in Hmong, our culture—no one else could see our Hmong women's private areas. Our husbands were the only people who could see in the middle of the night, without a single light on, our Hmong women's private areas. If I knew that the nurse or the doctor would like to see my private area today, I would not have come because I feel very ashamed to let someone else look at my private area. Our older Hmong people considered our private areas very personal and very sensitive areas to talk about. Back then, when our husbands and wives slept together, we slept at nighttime only. Our husbands and wives, we never wanted to see each other's private areas when there was still daylight because we felt that all adults should consider our private areas as secret or very personal private areas, and we should never talk about them in public or should never let someone else see them. There were probably only 1 percent of our Hmong women who slept with our husbands during the daytime, but the rest of us women never did because we were very shy. Mostly, our older Hmong women like me believed that if we let someone else see our private areas, then that means us Hmong women consider ourselves dirty people. In Laos, during the day times, the majority of our husbands never saw our Hmong women's private areas until the day we died. Interpreter, would you please tell the nurse that I will not let her or the doctor see my private area today. If they want to see it, I'd rather die.

Interpreter: (Interpreted exactly what the patient said to the nurse.)

Nurse: Okay, Dr. Anderson will be in shortly.

Interpreter: (Interpreted exactly what the nurse said to the patient.)

Doctor: (*Knocks*) I am Dr. Anderson. How are you today?

Interpreter: (Interpreted exactly what Dr. Anderson said to the patient.)

Patient: I already told the nurse that I did not want the doctor to touch my private area—period! Interpreter, can you please tell the doctor just do the general physical for me today only? Otherwise, if he wants to see it, I would rather want to leave now. Again, I do not want the doctor to touch my breasts or my private area at all. When I came to America, I heard a lot of my cousins and friends told me that American doctors do not mind to touch women's private areas and breasts when they do their physical examinations, but for me I do not want that kind of physical. If I knew that they wanted to see my private area today, I would have canceled my appointment yesterday, but I did not know. I know that doctor only wants to help me, but I do not like someone else to touch my private area and breasts at all. If I have any pains later, then I do not mind, but I do not feel any pain now at all; so I think it is not necessary to check it, right? I only allow my husband to touch and see it, and no one else can. Please forgive me.

Interpreter: (Interpreted exactly what the patient said to the doctor.)

Analysis for Case No. 2: Private Areas

It is a culture shock for the older Hmong woman patient because she never had any physical examination, including Pap smear, done in Laos before. Since she never heard the word "Pap smear" before and never knew what a Pap smear meant exactly to her, so the moment she heard the word "Pap smear," in which the doctor would use a special plastic device to go inside a female's vagina to see if there was a cancer or not, she did not feel comfortable at all in allowing the doctor to do it. The moment she heard the nurse describe the definition of Pap smear to her, she then rejected the idea quickly.

In the Hmong culture back in Laos, our Hmong people never had any physical examinations done before, so for this female patient, she felt very ashamed as to why the doctor and the nurse wanted to see her private area. Probably in her mind, she probably thought that they did not treat or respect her as an adult; that was why they asked to see her private area, like a little kid. Furthermore, she did not believe that having the Pap smear done was necessary since she was a healthy person. However, for us in the American culture in the medical field, every woman has to have an annual physical, including Pap smear. The reason we have to do an annual physical and Pap smear is to detect early signs of cancer in the cervical area or breasts. This would then allow the doctors to treat the disease early before it is too late.

Case No. 3: Killer Pills

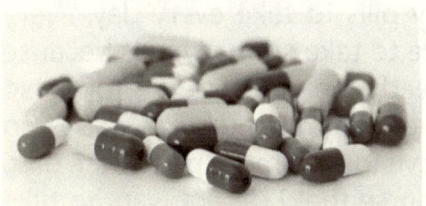

Patient: Ntxawm Ntxuaj Pag (seventy-one-year-old female patient)

Interpreter: Niam Nkauj Zuag Paj

Nurse: Brenda

Location: At the hospital

(Phone Ringing)

Interpreter: Hi, my name is Niam Nkauj Zuag Paj, and my ID no. is 11211. I speak Hmong. When you are ready, please go head.

Nurse: My name is Brenda, and I am your nurse until 11:30 p.m. tonight. I just received the order from your doctor this morning, and here are the medications for you to take, okay. One pill for your blood pressure, one pill for your diabetes, one pill for your heart, one pill for your gout, and one pill for your lungs.

Interpreter: (Interpreted exactly what the nurse said to the patient.)

Patient: Every day when the nurse comes to check on me, she always wants me to take pills, pills, and pills! Why does the nurse keep giving me so many pills to take every day, every day, and every day? I do not like to take so many pills because they are not good for me. I already feel much better today, so I'm not taking any more pills. Every day, the nurse keeps saying the same thing to me—that I have to take more pills, more pills, and more pills. Please tell the nurse that I do not want to take them anymore. She needs to take them back where she got them from. Taking too many pills is bad for my body. Did the nurse remember that she gave me too many pills to take the last couple of days ago already? Some of the pills that the she gave to me were too strong and almost killed me. Now I am back to live; I refuse to take the pills. If I want to die, I want to die peacefully and will go to the sunshine road in heaven; so I will try to be that person, okay? That is why I refuse to take the pills.

Interpreter: (Interpreted exactly what the nurse said to the patient.)

Nurse: If you want to go home, you need to take these pills. These pills will help you get better. If you do not want to take them, you will have to stay in the hospital longer.

Interpreter: (Interpreted exactly what the nurse said to the patient.)

Patient: If the nurse keeps pushing me to take these pills, maybe the nurse wants me to die. I think maybe she does not want me to live anymore. Interpreter, please tell the nurse that if she makes me take these pills and I die, then I will never forget her. I already told her that these pills are bad for me because I took them several days ago, and they almost killed me. If I take them again today, I know I will die for sure because they are bad for me. Why didn't the nurse understand me? I will not take them because I still want to live! No matter what the nurse says, I will not take them because they are not good for me! Like I said earlier, I took them before, and I almost died! If she still wants to force me to take the pills, I will close my mouth. Or if she puts the pills in my mouth, I will spit them out.

Nurse: I want you to get better so that is why I give you these pills. If you want to get better, you have to take them. Okay, I will let your doctor know that you do not want to take them.

Analysis for Case No. 3: Killer Pills

In the Hmong culture, most of our older Hmong people believe that taking too much pills can kill us, and when we die from the pills it is considered poisoning. Poisoning is considered as suicide. In the Western culture, in order to get better, the sick patient must take the pills; but for our Hmong culture, taking too many pills is harmful. For Hmong patients, medications can be considered very dangerous to them, so if American doctors and nurses do not take the extra time to explain through Hmong interpreters or translators until they understand, then Hmong patients will likely refuse to take pills like the case above.

In Laos, only rich people who lived in the big city could buy pills from the stores and took them when they were sick. For poor people who lived in the mountainous rural regions, when they were sick, most of the time, our older Hmong people believed that using earthy or natural medicine was better and safer, especially because their origins were known, as a result of being grown in the garden or they were naturally found in nature.

In our Hmong culture, it is also believed that if someone died of overdose of any kind of medicine, then he or she would go to heaven in the heavy rain, dark, and dirty roads, or the owner up in heaven would punish him or her and would never allow his or her spirit be reborn again. In the Hmong culture, most people very strongly believe that for those who die by natural sickness, they will go to heaven peacefully and walk on the sunshine road straight to their ancestors' world without frustration or struggle. However, for those who die of overdose of any kind of medication, they will face the dark road or the possible punishment by the Father of heaven.

For this particular older Hmong patient, the reason she refused taking the pills is because of her past experiences, belief, and different culture. She was scared that the pills would possibly harm her more and did not believe that the pills were helping her to get better. She was afraid that by taking too many pills, like the nurse asked her, she would probably end up overdosing on the pills. Given my understanding of Hmong culture, I would surmise that she was probably thinking that if she died, she would not get a chance to go to the sunshine road in heaven; thus, she refused to take the pills.

As the interpreter, I felt that the nurse's perspective was probably very frustrated. She was there to help the patient get better, but she did not understand why the patient was so against taking the pills because the pills would help ease her pain. When we do not understand the patients' thinking, and the patients do not see the nurse's point of view or purpose, there will definitely be feelings of frustration, misunderstanding, and lack of cooperation, thereby complicating the process of helping the patients to get well.

Case No. 4: Burning Bananas

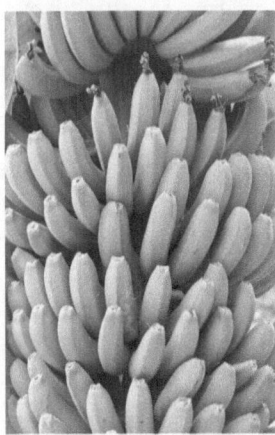

Patient: Paj Deg Liab (seventy-five-year-old female patient)

Triage nurse: Mary

Interpreter: Niam Nkauj Zuag Paj

Location: ER with Dr. Brown

(Phone ringing)

Interpreter: Hi, my name is Niam Nkauj Zuag Paj, and my ID no. is 11211. I speak Hmong. When you are ready, please go head.

Triage nurse: Hi there, my name is Mary, the triage nurse. I have a patient at the Emergency room right now. I need to ask her a question. "Why you are coming to the ER?"

Patient: Well, long ago, my family was still hiding at the jungle in Laos after the Vietnam War. I was probably about five or six years old, and I got very hungry. Since my family and I were so hungry, my father went to the forest and brought some of the green bananas to where the rest of my family was to eat. However, the bananas were still completely green and not ripe yet, so my mother told me and my siblings that we needed to burn the bananas on the fireplace until they were ready to eat; then we could eat. All of my brothers and sisters did exactly what my mother told us. After the bananas were completely burned from the fireplace and ready to eat, then we ate them. Every time when I ate something or did not eat anything after those green bananas, my stomach began to give me this terrible stomachache. Ever since I ate those burning bananas, my stomach started hurting me more and more than ever before. When we arrived in Thailand, my stomach was hurting several times again; but it did not hurt as much as now. Two days ago, I ate one banana in the afternoon for my snack, and after those two days, my pain started hurting days and nights. It was very painful, for I could not do anything around the house. I do not know why I have this pain for so long. I really want to get rid of it. Having this painful stomach problem—sometimes it makes me feel very depressed. Today, I decided to come to the ER to see the doctors to please help me. Why do I keep having this pain like this?

Interpreter: (Interpreted exactly what the patient said to the nurse.)

Triage nurse: Did you have any fever, throw up, or have any diarrhea at all?

Interpreter: (Interpreted exactly what the nurse said to the patient.)

Patient: Sometimes when it hurts a lot, then yes, I did have some fevers. When my fever became very bad—yes, I did throw up for a couple of times. I did not know why my stomach was hurting a lot, and even though I had this terrible stomachache, I had no diarrhea. I thought that if I was able to pass the bowel movements normally, then my stomach would feel a little bit better. But like I said, there was no diarrhea at all. Do you think that a banana can cause this painful stomachache too? I feel that it had to be something else that was causing this pain for so long inside of me.

Interpreter: (Interpreted exactly what the patient said to the nurse.)

Triage nurse: You may go back to the waiting room and wait for the nurses to call you to go in one of the exam rooms, okay?

Back office staffs: (*One of the nurses from the ER rooms opened the side door and called Paj Deg Liab*) Please follow me; this way (*as she was walking to one of the exam rooms*). (*The minute they went into an exam room, the nurse asked the patient to sit on the exam bed. The nurse began to ask her a lot of questions again.*) What brings you to the ER? How long have you had this pain?

Interpreter: (Interpreted exactly what the nurse said to the patient.)

Patient: Like I said earlier to the nurse at the front desk—long ago, I ate a burning banana. And after I ate it, my stomach started hurting me like this. This pain had started since I was a little girl back in Laos, while my family and I were still hiding in the jungle after the Vietnam War. When my family and I arrived in Thailand, the pain came back several times. When we came to America, the pain was gone. I do not know why now I have this pain back. Two days ago, I ate one banana for my snack, and after that, the pain just came back like this until today.

Please help me to check my stomach to see what is wrong with my stomach for me.

Interpreter: (Interpreted exactly what the patient said to the nurse.)

Nurse: We have to wait for the doctor to come to talk you today and will find out why you have this pain, okay. It is a possible that if the pain continues like this, maybe we will have to do a test call the colonoscopy procedure. Maybe we have to draw some blood to check why you have this pain too?

Interpreter: (Interpreted exactly what the nurse said to the patient.)

Patient: What is a colonoscopy procedure? And why you have to draw some blood for what? I hate needles. I never like them. Last time I was at the hospital, and the nurses kept coming and drawing so much blood of me. When they drew the blood, they kept poking my both arms, and they hurt so much; so I refused to have blood test. If I am a nurse like them, I would like to poke them to see if they can feel the pain like me too. I do not know if they ever get poking from needles or not, but poking by needles they are hurting a lot.

Interpreter: (Interpreted exactly what the patient said to the nurse.)

Nurse: The colonoscopy procedure is to use a very small light attached to a long thin cord through your anus into your stomach to see why your stomach is having this pain.

Interpreter: (Interpreted exactly what the nurse said to the patient.)

Patient: You know what. No, I do not want that colonoscopy procedure. I think that if you are going to put that little light attaching to a very small cord into my bottom then I think it would be more painful after the procedure, right?. When we used to live in Laos, we never had to do such thing like that before; so I am very scared and refused to do it. What happen if the light and the cord possible could scratch the inside of my stomach, and it could be more damage and hurt more inside of me? The pain would never disappear and could only get worse. Are you sure that the doctor will know for sure that he will guarantee to me that he will not create more pain for me? Are you sure the doctor will not scratch the inside of my stomach?

Interpreter: (Interpreted exactly what the patient said to the nurse.)

Nurse: Well, again, we will have to do what your doctor wants us to do to help you. Maybe we just need to draw blood first and will do the procedure test later.

Interpreter: (Interpreted exactly what the nurse said to the patient.)

Patient: I do not know and understand why American doctors always want to draw so many tubes of patients' bloods when patients come to the hospital. I just wonder what do the nurses and doctors do with the patients' bloods. I think that if the doctors and nurses need to do just the blood test only then maybe a only few drops of blood to do the test, but I do not know why they have to draw so many tubes of bloods for what. Since I had this stomach problem, I could not eat much and probably did not have enough blood inside of me either; so I do not want the nurses to draw so much of my blood. Interpreter, please tell the nurses and doctors that I can allow them to draw just one tube of my blood only. I want them to know that I do not like needles at all too. Many years ago, I came to this hospital, and the nurses came to draw blood on me; and the nurse was probably very new worker at the hospital tried to poke me so many times before she could draw my blood. This time please poke only one time to draw my blood.

Interpreter: (Interpreted exactly what the patient said to the nurse.)

Nurse: Okay, just continue lying down on the bed. Today, we are very busy, so as soon as the doctor finishes seeing other patients, the doctor will come to see you.

Analysis for Case No. 4: Burning Bananas

This older Hmong patient was very frustrated with the nurse and the doctor because she already explained very clearly about the situation—how she got sick—to them, but the way they were talking to her seemed like they did not understand how she got sick at all. She did not realize that in the medical field when a patient had a stomachache there could be anything that caused the pain, so in order for the doctor to know exactly how to treat the patient's stomachache, he had to do a blood test or even a procedure called colonoscopy to see the inside of the stomach and what caused the pain exactly. From the doctor's point of view, since the patient had this pain for a long ago, maybe the patient could have an ulcer, or a tumor which may be cancerous. But for the patient, she just wanted to know why she had this pain. She knew very well that she ate the burnt banana long ago, and since then, her stomach began to hurt so she was hoping to have some pain medication to take care of it. On the other hand, in order for the doctor to give her the medication, the doctor first had to know exactly what kind of pain it was or what caused the pain.

For the colonoscopy procedure, after the nurse explained to her, she was so afraid that they would create more pain for her. She also did not believe that drawing blood to check the inside of her was necessary because she knew herself better; her stomach pain had nothing to do with the blood, and needles were also her enemy. As the interpreter, I could see that the nurse and the doctor were very frustrated because whatever they suggested to help her, the patient kept refusing to do what they recommended. This case is another example of a cross-cultural misunderstanding.

Case No. 5: The Traumatic Ear

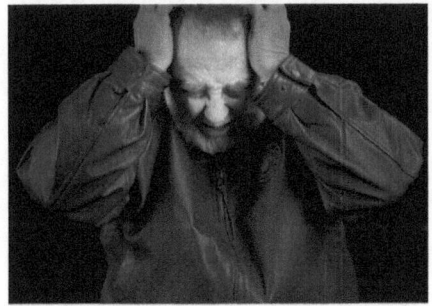

Patient: Txiv Nuj Sis Loob (seventy-six-year-old male patient)

Interpreter: Niam Nkauj Zuag Paj

Social Worker: Linda

Location: Hospital

(Phone ringing)

Interpreter: Hi, my name is Niam Nkauj Zuag Paj, and my ID number is 11211. I speak Hmong, and when you are ready, please go ahead.

Social Worker: Hi, my name is Linda, and I am a social worker. I have a patient with me here at the hospital now by the name of Txiv Nuj Sis Loob. He speaks just a little bit of English only so can you please help me talking to him. I think this patient has PTSD because earlier, he was trying to tell me something about the American CIA to me, but I did not understand him much. Interpreter, can you please ask him to please tell me why he is coming to the hospital?

Interpreter: (Interpreted exactly what the social worker asked the patient.)

Patient: I used to help the American (CIA) to fight with the North Vietnamese during the Vietnam War in Laos. I was one of the Hmong men who shot the big automatic guns to the Ho Chi Minh Trail Road, so North Vietnamese soldiers would not able to entrance to Laos. No matter how was the weather, cold or hot, sunshine, or rain at the jungle, my duty was to continue to shot at the Ho Chi Minh Trail Road to stop the North Vietnamese to come. I had been shooting the big automatic guns for many years in the most bombed city on earth called Xiang Khouang until 1975. After 1975 the American (CIA) left Laos, many other Hmong soldiers and I ran to hide at the jungle without our families because we over heard from our neighbors said that if the North Vietnamese soldiers ever found out that we helped the American (CIA) then they would kill us. One night it was raining very hard and too dark to see on the ground clearly. The rest of the Hmong soldiers and I were running away and climbing to the top of the tallest mountain in Laos which it called Phou Bia to find a safe place to sleep at. On that dark night, somehow I could not see very well in the forest because we had no flash lights, so I accidentally fell off from a very high place to the ground and hit my right ear on an old truck of tree and also small rocks around it too. On that night, I could not sleep at all because it was painful inside my right ear. On the next day, I continued to feel the terrible pain in my ear and also was bleeding a little bit from the inside. Again, there were no medications or doctors available to help us at the jungle, so I used nothing for the pain. All I did was to concentrate how to survive, and did not have time to concentrate about my ear. Two months later, the other Hmong men and I came back to our previous towns and found our wives and children there. We took our families and escaped to Thailand. When we arrived to Thailand, my right ear was still hurting. One of the most well known refugee camps where my family and I stayed at was called Ban Vinai Camp; I went to see a doctor at a local clinic. The doctor said that they had to do some minor surgery on my right ear and also gave me some medications to take by mouth. After that visit, I came home and took the medications. However, the pain was still there. I finally decided to have the surgery done. After the surgery, I was so happy that there was no more pain. In 1983, my family and I came to America. When we arrived in American, I did not know why something else came from my right ear. Every night, I started hearing noises like gun shots and people's voices from far away inside my right ear. These noises and voices were making me go crazy, especially at night. Since I have not been able to sleep very well, I have begun to have terrible headaches in the last couple of days. Especially today, I feel like my head is going to explode.

Social worker: Have you ever seen a counselor for your PTSD at a mental health clinic before?

Interpreter: (Interpreted exactly what the social worker said to the patient.)

Patient: Yes, I did. I went only two times, and I felt that it was a wasting time for me because I did not see how the counselors or psychiatrists could help me, so I stopped from going. I felt that they did not know how to help me much. What they did was continuously talking and giving me the medications only? To me, I did not feel they were helping me at all.

Social worker: It is a long procedure for people who had PTSD to recover. I encourage you to go back to see the counselors and psychiatrists if you can. They will help you to talk about your past and understand what you had been through, and if they feel that you will need different kind of medications to help you then they will give them to you. In order for you to get better, you have to take the medications that they gave you. If you do not take the medications, you will not get better sooner.

Interpreter: (Interpreted exactly what the social worker said to the patient.)

Analysis for Case No. 5: The Traumatic Ear

In this case, the social worker definitely thought that the older veteran Hmong male patient was dealing with PTSD as a result of his war experience. However, as for the patient, he did not understand what PTSD was, how it is treated, or how PTSD related to the physical ear pain he experienced. In this case, the social worker did his or her job correctly to help the patient, by suggesting to him that he needed to continue seeing the counselor and psychiatrist regularly in order to get the care that he needed. This included mental and physical support and also providing him with some medications that he needed to reduce his trauma, depression, or anxiety so he could feel better.

Case No. 6: Silent Birth

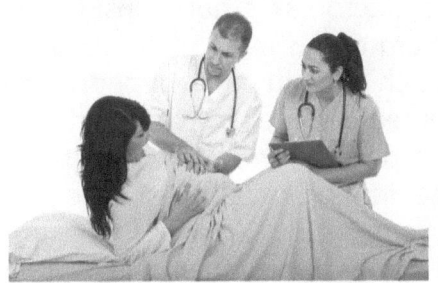

Patient: Ntxhais Ntiaj Teb (thirty-year-old female patient who just came from Laos recently)

Interpreter: Niam Nkauj Zuag Paj

Nurse: Susan

(Phone ringing)

Interpreter: Hi, my name is Niam Nkauj Zuag Paj, and my ID no. is 11211. When you are ready, please go head.

Nurse: My name is Susan, and I am a nurse at the hospital in the delivery room with a patient who is going to give birth very soon now, but I cannot communicate with her because she does not speak much English. Can you please help me ask her to see if her water broke yet?

Interpreter: (Interpreted exactly what the nurse said to the patient.)

Patient: No, my water is not broke yet. Interpreter, I want to share something with you. In Laos, I gave birth to my first and second children without a doctor or a nurse inside my home. While I gave birth to them over there, my aunt came and helped me delivery my two children in my own bedroom. Before I came to America, I overheard some people said that if the unborn child is too big then possible the doctor will have to cut the mother's private area little bit bigger and wider, so the baby can come out easily. Is that true? Also, many of my friends told me that when all mothers had their children at the hospital the doctors and nurses would not let all mothers doing the duckling styles while they were giving birth. I want to tell you and the nurse right now that when it is time for me to give birth to my baby then I will have to do what I did in Laos to give birth to my child. I will not follow the doctors or nurses' orders how to give birth to my child because according to my own experience by giving birth the way that our Hmong mothers and myself did in Laos were much faster and easier. I will never forget what my mother said to me, "Listen! During your pregnancy, you must keep working, working, and working inside the house or at the field until the last minutes that you know you are going to give birth soon then you can stop working. You cannot lie down all day long and sit all day to keep waiting to give birth. When you are lay down all day long and keep waiting to give birth to your child only and do nothing then when it is time to delivery it is going to be a very difficult for you and the baby. If it is getting very close to your due date, and the contractions start beginning, you must not lay down on the bed only. You must still walk around the house and get ready to find a comfortable place to give birth like in the bedroom. When you start realizing that the contractions are coming so close to each other then you must go to your bedroom and do the duckling style next to the bed and ready to give birth. If you do nothing during your pregnancy and just sit all day long to wait for the baby to come out, the baby will take a long time to come out." For example from my past experience, through all my pregnancies, I walked every day to the field and worked all day long around the house. When I was about to give birth to my two older children in Laos, the moment that I started having the contractions between three to five minutes apart then I went to my bedroom quickly and began to do my duckling styles nearby my bed to kneel down as I was about to give birth. From my both past experiences, the minutes I found myself comfortably on the floor holding the corner of the bed then I would become to do my duckling styles as soon as I could without moving around then a few moments later I gave birth to my babies. I realized that in this way I did not have to push so hard if I did not lying down on my back on the bed like the Americans' way at the hospital then the babies would come out much faster for me. During the whole time of my two previous deliveries from started to ended, I only had the contractions for a couple of hours, then my babies popped out. I believed that I took my mother's advice and gave birth to my children so quickly, and also because I worked all of the time at the field every day up-down everywhere without taking a single day off during my pregnancies, so that was why I gave birth to them so fast.

Interpreter: (Interpreted exactly what the patient said to the nurse.)

Nurse: Okay, that is fine.

Patient: My mother used to tell me that if I wanted my baby to be born fast then when my contractions began I should never yell or scream at all because if I yelled or screamed very loud while the contractions were coming then the baby would not come out right away. When my contractions were coming, I should be silence without making a single noise and just breathed quietly only as the contractions came; so my baby could come out faster. Otherwise, in our Hmong culture, we believed that if the mothers yelled and screamed very loud while she was having the contractions then the baby would think that the mothers would not ready for the baby to come out yet because the mothers were still too busy singings.

Interpreter: (Interpreted exactly what the patient said to the nurse.)

Nurse: Can I check you again?

Interpreter: (Interpreted exactly what the nurse said to the patient.)

Patient: I do not understand why in America the nurses like to check us women's private areas so much when us women are having so much pain like right now. Since I came to the hospital, the nurse asked me to see my private area like about six times already. I just wonder how many more times the nurses will have to check my private area from now no? Interpreter, you know us Hmong women do not let anyone else see our private areas, right? Sometimes I did not feel comfortable for the nurses to check me that much.

Interpreter: (Interpreted exactly what the patient said to the nurse.)

Nurse: I have to check her consistently, so I will know exactly how many centimeter her vagina is dilated or not?

Interpreter: (Interpreted exactly what the nurse said to the patient.)

Patient: In our culture, we never check our Hmong women's private areas at all. When it is time for the baby to come out, he/she will naturally come out automatically without keep checking, right? To me, I do not believe that it is necessary to check so much like the nurse who is checking on me right now.

Interpreter: (Interpreted exactly what the patient said to the nurse.)

Nurse: I understand, but I have to follow the rules at the hospital and have to do what I have to do. Right now, it is a time for me to check her again. Okay, after I check her and if it is almost times, I will call the doctor right away.

Interpreter: (Interpreted exactly what the nurse said to the patient.)

Patient: Can I push now? I feel like pushing now!

Interpreter: (Interpreted exactly what the patient said to the nurse.)

Nurse: Don't push yet. She needs to wait little bit more because it is not time yet.

Interpreter: (Interpreted exactly what the nurse said to the patient.)

Patient: No! I cannot wait any longer! I know myself better than she?! When it is time to push, I have to push!

Analysis of Case No. 6: Silent Birth

Different cultures use different techniques when it is time to deliver a baby. It was a very interesting case that this Hmong mother used to give birth to her other children without a nurse or a doctor back in Laos, and she did not realize how different it is in America when she had her third child. This female Hmong patient who just came from Laos to America did not understand how much different the Western culture was when it was time to give birth to a child. This Hmong mother who has given births twice in Laos, without the help of a doctor or a nurse, wanted to give birth in the same way. She never experienced a nurse or a doctor consistently checking up on her during the contraction times, and therefore, the checking system became a very confused and very uncomfortable experience for her during her delivery in the hospital. She did not realize that there were so many certain hospital rules for the doctors and nurses, who had to do their jobs correctly in order to best help the patient give birth to her new child safely.

The Hmong mother, who was concentrating very hard on her contractions, felt very frustrated that the nurse kept asking and checking on her cervix and telling her when not to push, based on how dilated her cervix was. For the Hmong mother, she was completely listening to her body telling her when it was time to push. This case demonstrates the need to be proactive about understanding and dealing with differences in cultural practices, such as giving birth. If we wait to deal with situations like this until the moment or event, everyone will experience a great deal of stress.

Case No. 7: Hospital Sleepover

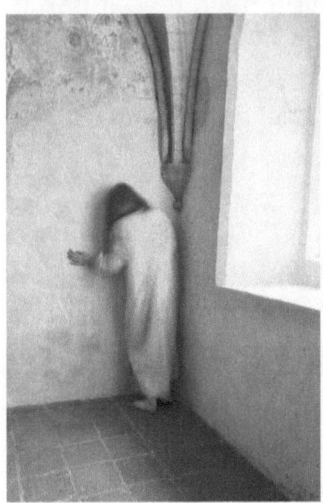

Patient: Maiv Paj Tsw Qab (ninety-year-old female patient who had a very difficult time hearing)

Nurse: Nancy

Interpreter: Niam Nkauj Zuag Paj

Hospital: Patient's room

(Phone ringing)

Interpreter: Hi, my name is Niam Nkauj Zuag Paj and my ID number is 11211. When you are ready, please go ahead.

Nurse: Hi, my name is Nancy. I am a nurse who will be taking care of Maiv Paj Tsw Qab tonight. Can you tell me your name, and how old are you, where are you at, and what date is today?

Interpreter: (Interpreted exactly what the nurse said to the patient.)

Patient: Young girl, young girl, are you a Hmong lady right? Can you speak louder because I cannot hear you that well? What did you just say? You said that you are coming to visit me? Yes, can you come right now? I am very scared to stay here alone. I don't know where are my children and grand-children at? Why no Hmong people here with me? Last nights, I saw ghosts in this room with me. They were watching me all night long over there at that corner. They kept smiling at me, and I even saw some of them climbed on to my bed, and sat next to me. I kept yelling, yelling, and yelling at the nurses to come and sleep with me, but they never came. I think that these American doctors and nurses are not nice people and have very black hearts because they did not want to help me at all. This morning when I woke up, I was very hungry, and they did not bring any food for me to eat either; so I do not want to stay here any longer and want to go home now. But, if the doctor still wants me to sleep here, young girl, can you please come here, sleep with me, and talk to me tonight. If you will not come in tonight, I don't know what I will do. You must come to see me because I will go home tomorrow; you will not see me anymore. When you come, can you please bring some Hmong food for me because I am very hungry?

Interpreter: (Interpreted exactly what the patient said to the nurse.)

Nurse: I am very sorry to hear that. I want you to know that I cannot come to your room and stay with you all night because I have many other patients who are waiting for me to take care of them too. I will do my best to take care of you, okay.

Analysis of Case No. 7: Hospital Sleepover

In this case, as the interpreter, I recognized that there were multiple factors that would complicate communication. First of all, this older Hmong patient appeared to have a very difficult time hearing me, maybe as a result of loss of hearing. Secondly, she appeared to be confused about questions—perhaps a sign of dementia. For example, when the nurse asked her many questions about who she was and where she was, she did not respond at all. Lastly, she did not seem to understand at all how the hospital's system works. She kept asking for the nurse to sleep with her because she was scared. Clearly, she did not know that in the hospital, the nurses could not sleep in the same room with her; they had to take care of many other patients.

She thought that the hospital was just like being at home. Whoever came to visit her could stay and sleep with her in the same room. She even asked me, the interpreter, if I could come and stay with her too. Despite the fact that her request for someone to come sleep next to her as a companion probably could not be delivered; it was interesting that the nurses just dismissed her. The patient kept on reporting that she was afraid because she sees ghosts in the building—an indication it is haunted. Maybe they thought she was hallucinating and didn't take it seriously. However, in the Hmong culture, it is believed that there are spirits everywhere, and sometimes they are not good spirits and can have ill intentions, causing someone to become very sick. This phenomenon, if not attended to or taken seriously, can cause a person to experience spiritual loss.

Case No. 8: Water Medicine

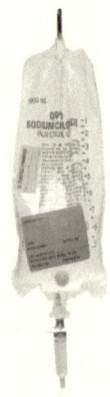

Patient: Txiv Nraug Sis Nab (seventy-eight-year-old male patient)

Nurse: Tom

Interpreter: Niam Nkauj Zuag Paj

Hospital: Patient's room

(Phone ringing)

Interpreter: Hi, my name is Niam Nkauj Zuag Paj, and my ID number is 11211. When you are ready, please go ahead.

Nurse: My name is Tom. I am Txiv Nraug Sis Nab's nurse at the hospital. It seems like he is trying to tell me something, but I did not understand him at all. Can you please help me find out what he needs?

Interpreter: (Interpreted exactly what the nurse said to the patient.)

Patient: I know for sure that I have ulcer because my parents told me so. They explained to me long ago that if I ever felt the pain right below my ribs inside my stomach like right now then that was considered ulcer. Since I had this pain all the time, I could feel the pain was located exactly in the area where my parents told me; so that is why I said I have ulcer. Interpreter, please help me! The moment I came to this hospital, my stomachache is hurting me so much, so I am telling the nurse to give me the medication for me to take; but I don't know why the nurse did not understand me at all. I want the nurse to give me the same medication that I bought from the stores for me to take here because I know that the medication I used to take it at home it worked for me very well. I know that the hospital should have this kind of medication inside this huge hospital building. All hospitals should have all kind of medications available all of the time for their patients to take. I do not want to take any other kind of medications beside the one I used to take because I do not know if I take the other kind of medications would help my ulcer, so I just want to take the same kind that I used to take at home. Let me explain about the medication that I used to take for my ulcer at home to the nurse, so she will know exactly what medication I am talking about it. The bottle is not too big, and it is round kind. The medication inside the bottle is pink. If she goes to the store, the medication is everywhere on the shelves. She is a nurse, so she should know the medication I am talking about. Interpreter, can you please tell the nurse to please bring the same kind medication that I just explain to her to me?

Interpreter: (Interpreted exactly what the patient said to the nurse.)

Nurse: I just gave him a pain medication not too long ago, so it is not time for the second one yet. I need to know the name of the medication that he had at home, so I can check in the hospital to see if we have here. Please tell him that the medication that I gave him earlier was liquid medication, and it went through his IV; so he had to wait.

Interpreter: (Interpreted exactly what the nurse said to the patient.)

Patient: I don't think that the nurse gave me any medications at all. If she did, my pain should reduce less pain by now. I saw she only added water into the plastic bag and not medication. I want to take the pill medications. I know that the pills work faster and better for me and not the clear liquid. I don't think the American doctors and nurses really want to take care of me because whatever I asked them they refused to do. When my ulcer got very bad, I called my primary physician and made appointment to see him; but I had to wait for a very long time before I could go and saw him. If I continue to wait for a very long time to see my doctor like in the past, the next time I will probably die before my appointment. Every time when I picked up my medications, there were only one or two pills inside the bottle for me to take. To me, I felt that the pharmacist wanted me to die, so that was why he/she only gave one or two pills for me to take each time. Also at the hospital same thing, they refused to give me the pills that I asked to take because they just wanted me to die soon. I know my ulcer better than anyone else. I want them to give me the same medication that I used take at home, but they did not listen to me at all. Since I arrived to the hospital without taking the medications from home, I felt my stomach was getting worse and worse than ever before because I felt that there were so many gases inside of me. Even I passed gases through, my stomach is still hurting. Sometime my back is also hurting so much too. I don't know why my two feet were so swollen too. I know the reason why the doctors and nurses did not want to give me the good medications because they do not want me to live anymore, so they can open me up to practice to gain experience and knowledge for them. I want them to know that if they don't take a good care of me and let me die because they wanted to do the surgery on me. In Hmong culture, we believe that our ancestors will come and take them to heaven to punish them because they did not want to take a good care of me and let to me die.

Interpreter: (Interpreted exactly what the patient said to the nurse.)

Nurse: I will talk to the doctor to see he will order some more pain medications for his stomachache later today. No, we don't want him to die. We will help him to get better, so he can go home.

Interpreter: (Interpreted exactly what the nurse said to the patient.)

Patient: That is all I want to say. Thank you.

Analysis for Case No. 8: Water Medicine

The language barrier and different cultures are the main issues in this case. The nurse tried to get more information, but the patient only remembered the color of the medication that he took at home and nothing else. This made it more difficult for the nurse to find and give to him the same medication that he was taking at home. The patient felt frustrated that the nurse didn't know the medication he was talking about or trust that he knows what is going on with his body. From the nurse's point of view, she could not just give any kind of medication that patients ask for.

Besides a basic pain medication, the patient didn't realize that the nurse and/or doctor would have to diagnose his illness first before they would know exactly what medication to prescribe him. Such a situation led to the patient feeling like the nurses and doctors didn't want to or do not intend to truly help him. This was clearly a misperception. This case exemplifies cultural misunderstanding, conflict of cultural values, and different lens of the same issue: The nurse and doctor valued nonbiased information such as "we can help you, if you give us the name of the medication you were taking at home" vs. the Hmong patient who valued immediate results such as, "If you were truly helping me, my pain would subside."

Case No. 9: Interpreter Becomes the Patient

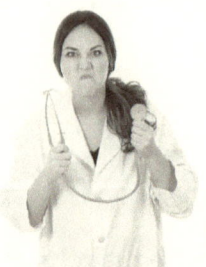

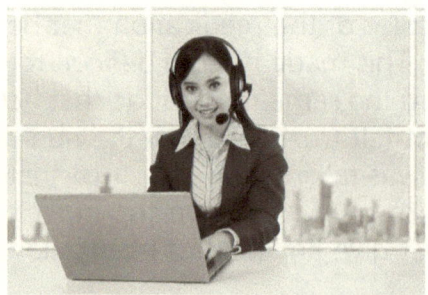

Patient: Maiv Paj Yeeb (eighty-nine-year-old female patient)

Nurse: Nue (She has a very heavy accent in her voice.)

Interpreter: Niam Nkauj Zuag Paj

Location: Hospital

(Phone ringing)

Interpreter: Hi, my name is Niam Nkauj Zuag Paj, and my ID number is 11211. When you are ready, please go ahead.

Nurse: My name is Nue. I am a nurse who is taking care of the patient by the name Maiv Paj Yeeb. Interpreter, I want you to interpret for me. I want to know how is the patient doing tonight, is she feeling better or does she have any pain now? Where is your pain level? Show me your pain, or can you point to it? Can you give me a number from zero to ten?

Interpreter: (Interpreted exactly what the nurse said to the patient.)

Patient: Interpreter, can you help me? I just came from the big tunnel downstairs, and I am very scared. While I was inside that huge tunnel, I thought I was going to die because I was having a hard time breathing in there. All my children probably went home already because they needed to go to work tomorrow, so I was having so much pain, could not talk to the nurse, and tried very hard to use my hands to communicate with the nurse to bring me some medications, but the nurse did not understand me at all. This nurse should know that I am having so much pain, so that was why I was ending up at the hospital, but it seemed like she did not care what I was trying to tell her.

She should know that I do not speak any English. Even I did not understand much English, I can tell that she kept saying a lot to me, but she never listened to me and brought me the medications. I do not want to talk to this nurse anymore because she is not an American nurse, and she is not nice like those American nurses that came last year. This time, I have a hard time understanding her because of her heavy accent. When she came to my room, she did not say hi or smile at all. Since she is not a very nice person, I cannot talk to her; I feel very depressed because I cannot say what I want to say to her. My pain is all over my body right now. Especially my ribs and chest are hurting a lot. I explained to her that I wanted some pain medications early today, but she pretended that she did not hear me.

Interpreter: (Interpreted exactly what the patient said to the nurse.)

Nurse: Interpreter, interpreter, I want to know what she said and what you interpret to the patient, and why she did not answer any of my questions. You need to interpret words to words. I do not think you interpret correctly because I can tell that the patient was saying a story; but you only said a few words to me. I want you to ask the patient again to answer all my questions that I asked you earlier. I want you to say exactly what the patient said, so you need to think back and interpret exactly what she said to me?

Interpreter: (Interpreted exactly what the nurse said to the patient.)

Patient: This nurse is a bad nurse because she did not listen to me at all and did do what I asked her to. I will not answer her because she refused to bring me the pain medications to me. Interpreter, can you tell her to stop asking and talking to me? Can you tell her that every time when I came to this hospital in the past, all of the nurses were very nice to me, but this time this nurse is not nice at all? I will not talk to the nurse because she is wasting my time to talk to her.

Interpreter: (Interpreted exactly what the patient said to the nurse.)

Nurse: Interpreter, are you sure you interpret right because the patient did not answer my questions. I want to know if she has bowl movement today at all or not. Is she ever having Hepatitis B and TB test in the past? If she did have them before, where did she get treat at?

Interpreter: (Interpreted exactly what the nurse said to the patient.)

Patient: Again, like I said earlier, I want my pain medications. Can you tell her I will not answer her questions unless she brings the medications to me because she already asked me these same questions yesterday? I am very tired to answer her same questions. If she continues asking these same questions next time again I will go hide away from her she is not a good nurse to me. If I had Hepatitis B and TB test done before, I was probably death by now. Every time when I got sick, I always went to see my doctor, so my doctor should know what I have. Since she is a nurse, she should know who my doctor is. She knows how to read and write, so she should know where my doctor's office and what my doctor's phone number are.

Interpreter: (Interpreted exactly what the patient said to the nurse.)

Nurse: Do you know you name? Where are you now? What date is today? Can you tell me what month is this month? Who is your doctor? Do you know your doctor's phone number?

Interpreter: (Interpreted exactly what the nurse said to the patient.)

Patient: I can't read or write, so I do not know who my doctor is or his phone number. All I know is that he is an American doctor, and his office is over there. When I went to see my doctor at his office, then my children drove me over there; and they took me on a big road. I heard they said while we were driving on the big road that we took off on freeway 84 north sides and went straight to his office. If she goes outside right now, she should look for the tallest tree in town then that was where my doctor's office was locating at. There were Save-Mart Super Market, Dollar Tree stores, and Chinese restaurant next to his office. Interpreter, I want you to know that I do not want to stay at the hospital anymore because I can tell that this nurse is not an honest person, so I want to go home tomorrow. In the past, when I came to the hospital, all nurses were very nice to me not like this one.

Analysis for Case No. 9: Interpreter Becomes the Patient

In this case, I did not know what caused the patient to be so angry at the nurse. The minute I begin to interpret for the nurse and the patient for the very first time, the patient was already very angry at the nurse. I think the reason why the patient did not answer her questions was because the nurse did not do what this non–English-speaking Hmong patient wanted, and she did not realize that the patient was already very upset at her.

Furthermore, she continued to repeat too many questions for the patient to answer, and that was why the patient got so mad and refused to talk to her. As a result, the nurse was accusing and blaming me that I was the one who did not know how to interpret correctly for the patient to understand; so that was why the patient never answered her questions. I felt that the nurse should have listened to the patient's complaints rather than focusing the blame on me. If the patient had felt that the nurse understood her, than perhaps she would have answered her questions.

Case No. 10: Death and Dying

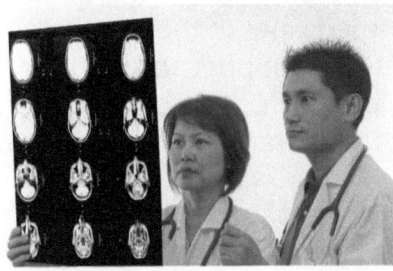
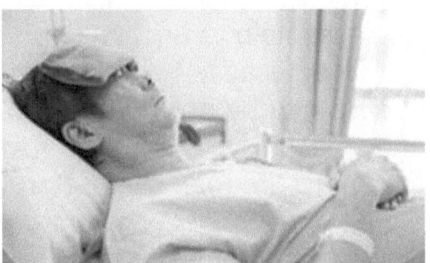

Patient: Npuag Txos Muaj (eighty-one-year-old male patient)

Interpreter: Niam Nkauj Zuag Paj

Location: At the hospital with Dr. Cooper

(Phone ringing)

Interpreter: Hi, my name is Niam Nkauj Zuag Paj, and my ID number is 11211. When you are ready, please go ahead.

Doctor: I am Dr. Cooper at the hospital. I am here in the room with a patient by the name of Npuag Txos Muaj. Npuag Txos Muaj, I need to talk to you and your family regarding your current situation. I have been treating you for quite a while now, and nothing seems to be working for you. I have been trying every medicine at the hospital that I know of to help you, but nothing works. There is no other way for me to help you get any better because the liver cancer that you have is already destroying your other organs very badly, and there is nothing much for me to do at this point.

Interpreter: (Interpreted exactly what the Doctor said to the patient and his family.)

Patient: Interpreter, can you please help me to tell the doctor to please help to find other better medicines in the hospital to help me because I want to get better. I suppose to get better in each day by now, but I do not know why I become weaker and weaker every day, and just a few days ago I notice that I feel more tire than ever before.

Doctor: There are two options that I would like to discuss with you and your family today. Since your situation is not getting any better, we need to prepare you to transfer to either hospice which it is also considering like a nursing home for you to keep you comfortable there, or if your family wants, you can go home; and we can send a nurse to come to check on you once a week or twice a week making sure you are comfortable. Otherwise, a patient who has a situation like yours cannot continue staying at the hospital any longer. We are thinking and planning to transfer you to the hospice place or at home probably by two next weeks, ok.

Interpreter: (Interpreted exactly what the doctor said to the patient.)

Patient: I do not want to go home or go to a nursing home yet because I have no energy at all, so I still want to stay here for the doctor to help me to get better before I will go home. Please let me stay in the hospital longer until I can walk by myself than I will go home. I do not want to get sick; I want to get better, so I can go home. But, I do not know why I keep feeling very tired lately. I know myself well very that if I am this weak like right now, and I go home, how I can walk around the house. (*Then patient's oldest son says*) I am his oldest son, and I really concern about his weakness. I know that he is so weak at this moment is because he cannot eat or drink at all. The reason he is able to talk right now is because the IV fluids which they help him a lot, so us children want him to continue to stay in the hospital to get more IV fluids until he feels better then we will take him home.

Interpreter: (Interpreted exactly what the patient and his oldest son said to the doctor.)

Doctor: I don't know what else I should say or explain to the patient and his family, so they can understand me. I am very sorry that I have to say what I have to say. The reason we have to transfer the patient is because he is not getting any better. He is getting weaker and weaker each day because his cancer is already spreading all over his body now, so that is why he is not eating and feeling very tired.

Patient: I do not want to go to the nursing home. I want to go home from here, but I cannot go now yet because I am still very tired. Can the doctor explain to me why I am so tired?

Interpreter: (Interpreted exactly what the doctor said to the patient and his family members, *but nobody seemed to understand what the doctor was saying about the patient's near-death situation. After our translation went back and forth for a little bit, and the doctor repeated their options several times, I realized that both parties were not on the same page. Neither the patient nor the family members realize the extent of the patient's medical situation, and in fact, this was a wait-until-death situation. I thought to myself, "What do I need to do now to help both parties?" I felt that the doctor needed to talk frankly with the family members in private about the patient's dying situation. Furthermore, I knew that I needed to share with the doctor the Hmong cultural beliefs and nuances of how to talk about the subject of death and dying. In Hmong culture, especially for the older Hmong generations, it is not appropriate or sensitive to tell someone who is near death that he/she is going to die.*)

Doctor: Again, I really do not know what else I can say to make sense to the patient and his family.

Interpreter: Doctor! I am very sorry to interrupt you, but I think it is best for us to continue discussing this issue in a separate room without the patient. Can we go to another room without the patient? *(One in a private room, I proceeded to share Hmong cultural values and beliefs about death and dying with the doctor.)* In our culture no matter how soon the patient will die, we cannot say straight to the patient yet that he is going to die because we do not want the patient to be sad, scared, and hopeless. We want to avoid the sadness for the patient. The reason I have asked everyone to go to another room is so we can talk very openly and very straight about how soon the patient will die rather than going around the bushes to the family members. You have already said several times there is nothing else you can do and the family members still do not appear to understand what you were exactly saying. Doctor, you and I have to say straight to the family members now that their father is going to die very soon because his cancer is getting very bad. I need to explain to them that they need to know their father is waiting to die now. He cannot continue to stay at the hospital because there is no medicine that will help. That is why he needs to go to the hospice. The other part of our culture is that especially when the patient is still alert and can understand what is happening around him, such as in this patient's case, we never want to tell the patient so directly that he is going to die. Not only will the fact that the end is near be too painful and too sad, it will break the sick person's heart that there is nothing else anyone can do and make him feel as though everyone has given up on him.

Doctor: Ok. *(Invites family members to the private room.)*

Interpreter: Doctor! Is everyone in the room now?

Doctor: Yes we are here.

Interpreter: (*I then begin to explain clearly what the doctor was saying to the family members.*) As you all heard in the room earlier, the doctor is trying to tell you children that your father is dying. His cancer is taking his life slowly at this moment; that is why he does not eat or drink any more. He is getting weaker and weaker each day because the cancer is all over his body. Right now he is just waiting to die. The doctor has tried all that he could to help your father but the cancer is too far along. He cannot stay much longer at the hospital; he needs to go to the hospice, which is a place where very sick people like him stay and wait to die. Or, if you children want, he can go home and stay with you children until the last day of his life. If he is at home, a nurse will come to see him twice a week to make sure he is comfortable while he is waiting to die. Like the doctor said early, he cannot do anything else to help your father anymore. The doctor thinks that your father will probably die very soon in the next couple of weeks.

Patient's family members: We understand much better now. Thank you for giving the information about exactly what is going inside our father's body and how critical his condition is. Today, there are still many of our family members who are not here with us, so we cannot make the decision yet. In Hmong culture, the whole family has to be here to make the decision. My father's youngest brother, who is coming from Laos, will be here in two days. So when he is here, we would like to have another meeting with this doctor before we will make the final decision. Can we set up another meeting for next Monday morning at 10:00 a.m. with this doctor again? Last question, can our father stay in the hospital for at least another week to see how he is doing before they will transfer him to the hospice or coming home because we want to make sure that he is doing a little bit better before he leaves the hospital?

Interpreter: (Interpreted exactly what the family's members said to the doctor.)

Doctor: Yes, he can stay in the hospital for another week.

Analysis for Case No. 10: Death and Dying

In this case, although my intervention helped both sides to come to a consensus, I could not fully help the doctor understand why death and dying is such a sensitive subject at the time, which would have required some extra time, patience and further explanation. But for anyone who will be dealing with these types of cases, it is imperative to have a deep understanding of how the Hmong people perceive death and dying.

In our Hmong culture, our older Hmong generations believe that when we die our dead bodies will rot underground, but our spirits will go to heaven. The Hmong words used to refer to heaven or the spirit world are *ntuj ceeb tsheej*. We believe that the spirits of all of our ancestors, families, and extended families—grandparents, parents, aunts, uncles, brothers, sisters, and relatives—will go to heaven and reunite until our spirits are reborn again. Our grandparents and parents believe that up in heaven, there is a very important person, Yawm Saub (a deity similar to or is God), who created everything visible and invisible around us—the Earth, heaven, sky, moon, sun, people, animals, nature, water, universe, and the spirit world. The majority of our older Hmong generations believe that Yawm Saub is in charge of taking care of our spirits before we are reborn on Earth. Our grandparents and parents believe that before a person is born to his/her parents on Earth, Yawm Saub will give him/her a paper of life, which describes his/her life on Earth, like a road map, including things like personality and gender.

We believe that Yawm Saub gives each of us a time of one hundred and twenty years to live on Earth before we die. The reasons some of us die before we reach one hundred and twenty years old are because of sickness, someone killing us, eating poisonous plants, dying of overdose, or other reasons that cause us to die sooner. If we die before reaching one hundred and twenty years, we will face the consequences by Yawm Saub. When our spirits go back to heaven, Yawm Saub will ask our spirits why and exactly how we died. If the reason for dying was because of sickness due to natural causes, Yawm Saub will not punish the spirit. Yawm Saub will let the spirit who died of sickness the choice and chance to be reborn back on Earth again. However, for those who died because of other reasons as mentioned above, the spirits will get punished for sure.

In the punishment process, our grandparents and parents believe that up in heaven, there are nine crossing roads. At each road, there are twelve gates with bodyguards at each of the main entrances for the spirits to pass through before the spirits meet with Yawm Saub. At the individual gates, there are bodyguards who will screen the spirits with questions like, "Why did you die?" "Did you kill someone?" "Did someone kill you?" "Did you poison yourself?" "Did you overdose on drugs?" Or, "Did you die as a result of a sickness?"

There are three main roads out of the nine crossing roads that spirits will have to face or take:

1. One is the sunshine road for those spirits who die of sickness. In this sunshine road, there are beautiful and colorful flowers everywhere on the ground along the road, greenish trees up the hills, mountains, and valleys, and birds are singing lovely songs just like on Earth until reaching the other peaceful world where Yawm Saub and all the ancestors', grandparents', parents', aunts', uncles', brothers', sisters', and close relatives' spirits live. When the spirits reach his/her immediate family members' spirits in the other world, they all can live happily until they are reborn back on Earth. If someone knows that they are dying from a natural illness, they are more at peace because they know that they will go on the sunshine road and then directly to their ancestors' home up in heaven.

2. The second road is the one for those who die from gunshots or any other violent weapons, grenade explosion, or murder. In this second road, the spirits will definitely face the consequences in a very unpleasant place, probably like a jail or detention, until the spirits are able to answer the tough questions correctly about how and why they died, then the spirits can go to the other world to be reborn again; otherwise, these spirits will stay there forever. Our grandparents and parents believe that Yawm Saub created us and made the decision for us to live peacefully on Earth, without fighting one another or killing someone. Anyone who died because of any of these violent weapons has to face punishment because he/she did not follow Yawm Saub's rules. Yawm Saub will tell the bodyguards to continue asking and questioning these spirits very closely in order for them to pass through each of the gates. If the spirits fail to answer the questions about why and how they died, Yawm Saub will not let these spirits be reborn. In order for these punished spirits to be released they must answer all the questions correctly. If they can't for whatever reason, it is believe that sometimes they may come back to make a family member ill and die in order to have that family member go help them. This may help release the punished spirit to be reborn again.

3. The third dark road, as characterized by heavy storms and dark clouds, is for those spirits who have died of an overdose on medicine such as opium or eaten poisonous plants. The spirits who died in this manner are usually walking on this scary, dark road alone. Meanwhile, inside their mouths are growing poisonous plants and a nonstop fill-up of opium juices and powdered medicine. These spirits are the ones who suffer for a very long time in heaven. Again, it is believe that sometimes these spirits will come back to cause a family member to become ill and die, so as to help them as stated above. If there is a situation where a spirit comes back to cause ill to the living family members, the first step or fastest way to appease the ill or evil spirit is to burn incenses and offer special spirit money to pay off the bodyguards to allow the spirit to go to the other

world. If the problem does not get resolved, then the family must ask a shaman to enter the spirit world and negotiate with the bodyguards and Yawm Saub to please allow the spirits to pass through the gates of heaven, without causing problem to the living family members. This process is usually accompanied by an animal sacrifice (chicken, pig, goat, or cow); these animals are believed to have extreme spiritual value and can appease spirit world.

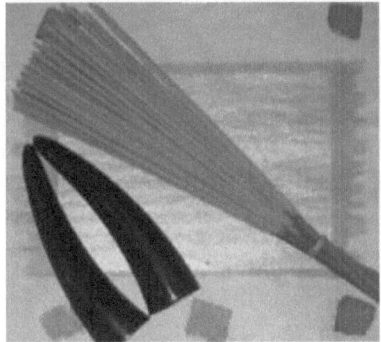

"Author's Own Photo": A sample of a bundle incenses and fake paper money to burn to the spirits.

Our older Hmong generations believe that in the last two roads of the nine crossing roads lay the most serious punishment for those who die of sickness. The consequences will not only affect the spirit's ability to be reborn for eternity, but will also affect the living family members who will have to deal with these bad spirits for possibly generations to come. This is why our older Hmong grandparents and parents are very scared of death, and everyone tries their very best to keep the family members healthy and good. Moreover, family members are very cautious and try to help family members from overdosing or eating any poisonous plants. Because of this uncertainty and the complicated process of the nine crossing roads before reaching the other peaceful world in heaven, the majority of our older Hmong people believe that dying is a very scary and lonely process.

In our culture, most older Hmong people still very much believe that even though we know for sure that a patient is going to die in the next couple of weeks, days, or hours, we still have to pretend in front of the patient that he/she will get better soon and must keep it a secret from the patient, because if the patient knows that he/she is going to die, then he/she can feel very sad, be hurt a lot, and cry a lot at the anticipated loss of his/her immediate families, lover, or children. We still want to ease the fear by telling the patient that he/she is going to get better soon and show the patient that we love and care for him/her very much, because we do not want him/her to know that he/she is going to die and will have to travel alone. This is true even up to the final moment of death.

It is not about being in denial. Everyone knows the reality of the situation. It is a way to show the person how much we love and care about him/her. The other reason is that if we are too direct with the patient who is going to die, then that means we do not love him/her; so that is why we do not want to tell him/her that he/she is going to die and watch him/her die without helping him/her. Even if we know that we cannot do anything to save him/her from dying, we still have to show him/her that we will ask the shaman to do everything within his or her power to stop the patient from dying. This is an emotional prolonging of the fact that death is near. This cultural understanding is important to know how this sensitive topic is discussed or framed in front of the patient. This is why when a Hmong patient is nearing death there are many families and extended family members by his or her side.

In reality, the immediate family members must know that the patient is dying, and it is important that the doctor is clear about expectations. For this particular cancer patient, after we went to another room, I explained very clearly to the family members, without the patient hearing, that their father is dying right now. Giving them the reason why their father could not stay any longer at the hospital because their father is just waiting to die. The cancer has already spread all over his body, and he will die very soon. I explained that they need to prepare for his death. What the doctor can do now is to let him stay in the hospital for a couple more days, then they have to transfer him to a hospice facility, or he can go home and a nurse will come to check on him to make sure he is comfortable. After we talked very openly about their father's critical condition, the family had to make the decision on what they wanted to do with their father's situation. After a whole hour of explanation about the process of their father dying, it seemed like they understood their father's situation better.

I have lived in America for almost forty years, and I pretty much understand what the word "dying" means in the American culture. I understand that when a doctor talks about dying, it means that the doctor knows to some extend when his patient is going to die within a certain time frame. Doctors will tell and say directly to the patient and the family how long or how soon the patient will die. The doctor will explain exactly how the patient is going to die to the patient himself/herself and the family members without hesitating. I believe that in the American culture there is a perspective that a person has only one life to live. Thus, doctors are direct with the patient and his/her immediate family members so that they will have enough time to say good-bye, to finish any unfinished business, or to get a chance to do something they wanted to do before the patient leaves this world forever. However, for our older Hmong generation, it is the opposite from the American culture. The word "death" for the older Hmong generation means that our physical bodies will never see again those we love. Thus, nearing death, the focus is on non-separation and comfort. Today, this can get complicated because the younger Hmong generation has adapted to the American culture. Within the Hmong community today, you have intergenerational differences in perspectives, beliefs, and ways of doing things—which could lead to misunderstandings, complications, or conflicts. Medical providers and other professionals who are sensitive to these things will have a better chance of working successfully with the Hmong patients.

Chapter Two

Effective Utilization of an Interpreter by American Medical Providers

There are many medical doctors, nurses, and other professional staffs who know what they need to do and how to utilize the interpreter in the right way. I find that the most effective way is when they ask one question at a time or say only a few words and then pause for the interpreter to interpret. This is known as consecutive interpreting. They need to recognize that they should not speak in long sentences or paragraphs without giving the interpreter the chance to interpret. In addition, the medical provider needs to know or ask for whom they should speak to in order to get certain information, understanding that the non–English-speaking Hmong patient does not know how to speak, read, and write in English. Sometimes it is their children or family members who know and have access to the information that they are seeking. Below are some cases that demonstrate the best practices and worst practices when using an interpreter.

Case No. 1: Turn-Taking Method (Consecutive Interpreting)

Patient: Tub Tuam Thawj (one-year-old boy)

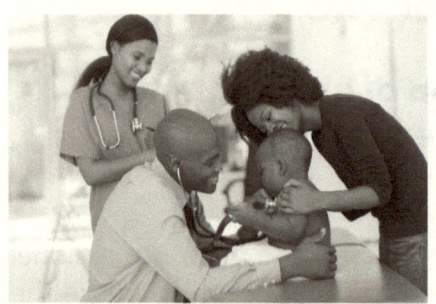

Nurse: Tracy

Location: Dr. Johnson's office

Interpreter: Niam Nkauj Zuag Paj

(Phone ringing)

Interpreter: Hi, my name is Niam Nkauj Zuag Paj, and my ID number is 11211. When you are ready, please go ahead.

Nurse: My name is Tracy, the nurse. We have a Hmong patient in the exam room, and it seems like the patient's Mom does not speak much English. I would like to know what is wrong with the baby.

Interpreter: (Interpreted exactly what the nurse said to the patient's Mom.)

Patient's Mom: My baby has very high fever and coughs a lot recently.

Interpreter: (Interpreted exactly what the Mom said to the nurse.)

Nurse: How many days did the baby have these syndromes? Did Mom give any over-the-counter medications to the baby?

Interpreter: (Interpreted exactly to the Mom what the nurse said.)

Patient's Mom: No, I did not. I did not know what kind of medications over the counter was good for my baby.

Interpreter: (Interpreted exactly what the Mom said to the nurse.)

Nurse: Okay, let me check the baby's temperature. Okay, the doctor will be in few minutes.

Interpreter: (Interpreted exactly what the nurse said to Mom.)

Doctor: (*Knocked on the door, then walked in.*) Hi, I am Dr. Johnson. Your baby has fever and cough. Did you try any over the counter medications yet?

Interpreter: (Interpreted exactly what the doctor said to Mom.)

Patient's Mom: No, not yet.

Interpreter: (Interpreted exactly what Mom said to the doctor.)

Doctor: Mom, can you please come and sit on this exam table and hold your baby on your lap? Let me exam your baby's body.

Interpreter: (Interpreted exactly what the doctor said to the Mom.)

Doctor: Your baby has an ear infection and cough, so I am giving you two prescriptions. One is the antibiotic for your baby's ear infection, and the other one is for your baby's cough, okay.

Interpreter: (Interpreted exactly what the doctor said to the Mom.)

Doctor: If your baby is not getting better while taking these medications in the next two weeks, please come back to see me again. Or if the baby is getting worse, please go to the ER as soon as possible, okay. The nurse will bring you the two prescriptions.

Interpreter: (Interpreted exactly what the doctor said to the Mom.)

Nurse: Okay, here are the prescriptions. Hope your baby will get better soon. Have a good day and bye.

Interpreter: (Interpreted exactly what the nurse said to the Mom.)

Analysis for Case No. 1: Turn-Taking Method (Consecutive Interpreting)

As the Hmong interpreter, I would say the case above was the most effective. The conversations were short and to the point. Each one of us knew exactly everyone's role and whose turn it was to speak. Each person did not say too little or too much, which I, as the interpreter, felt that it was easier to interpret back and forth. I enjoyed listening and talking back and forth between the patient, the nurse, and the doctor very much because the messages that we were passing onto one another on the phone were direct and clear. We learned to work together to make the patient feel that she was heard and her needs met; all of our needs were met. Everyone was satisfied and happy.

Case No. 2: All-at-Once Method
(Difficulty of Simultaneous Interpreting by Phone)

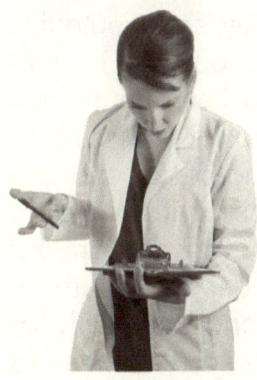

Patient: Maiv Nkauj Iab Oo (seventy-nine-year-old female patient who had all kinds of illnesses)

Nurse: Aurora

Interpreter: Niam Nkauj Zuag Paj

Location: Hospital

(Phone ringing)

Interpreter: Hi, my name is Niam Nkauj Zuag Paj, and my ID number is 11211. I speak Hmong. When you are ready, please go ahead.

Nurse: Hi, my name is Aurora, and I am the nurse who has been taking care of Maiv Nkauj Iab Oo.

The doctor said that you can go home today, so I would like to talk about the discharging instructions to you. First, I would like to start with all your medication then I will explain the rest of the information to you. Nothing changed for your current medication that you are used to taking at home, for example your Lovastatin, Metformin, and Allopurinol. Continue taking your Lovastatin 40 mg one tablet by mouth every day for your cholesterol; Metformin 1,000 mg one tablet daily by mouth for your diabetes; and take Allopurinol 300 mg one tablet daily for your gout. Here are the new medications that you will need to take. You will need to take these prescriptions to the pharmacy to get them on your way home, okay? The very first one is the antibiotic called Zithromax 250 mg—take two tablets by mouth daily for the first day and one tablet per day after that until it's all gone for your bladder infection. For your muscle back pain, take Hydrocodone 325 mg one to two tablets by mouth every four to six hours as needed. Take Fexofenadine 60 mg one tablet by mouth twice daily for your allergy and Indomethacin 50 mg one capsule by mouth three times daily with food for your arthritis. Lastly, take Tylenol with Codeine 25 mg one tablet by mouth for your back pain as needed. And you also have to use the following inhalers for your asthma when you are having any difficulty breathing. The kind of inhaler with the color blue—you only can use two puffs per day. For the pro-air inhaler, you only can use it four puffs per day. For the antibiotic medication, you have to take all of the pills until they are completely gone; you cannot just take the pills for a week and stop taking them. For the insulin, you have to poke your fingers daily before each meal to see if you need your insulin or not. You also need to follow up with your primary physician within a week. When you go see your primary physician, you have to take all these discharge papers with you to your doctor. However, if your situation is getting worse, you need to come back to the emergency room, ok? Do you have any questions regarding your medications? Do you understand everything I have said to you?

Interpreter: (*In this situation, I summarized as much information as I could to the patient.*)

Patient: Okay. No, I have no questions.

Interpreter: (Interpreted exactly what the patient said to the nurse.)

Nurse: Okay, if you understand the discharge instruction, please sign and date here. If you do not have any questions, I would like you to sign here and on the next page that you understand everything that I have said to you regarding the discharge instructions. After you are done signing all these pages, you can get dressed.

Analysis for Case No. 2: All-at-Once Method (Difficulty of Simultaneous Interpreting by Phone)

In contrast to case no. 1, a situation like this example above was absolutely the most difficult one for me as the interpreter, because the nurse did not pause in-between each sentence to allow me to interpret to the patient at all. It was only when she was completely done talking that she would let me take over the interpreting. In this case, it was impossible for me to interpret word for word from the nurse to the patient because there was too much information for me to remember. I felt that this was not good practice on the side or the nurse especially since this patient had to take so many different kinds of medications. In fact, it is quite dangerous, I believe. In my opinion, I think the nurse did a wonderful job explaining all of the details of the medications to the patient, but she needed to slow down to allow me to interpret the instructions in parts rather than in its entirety, to make sure the patient fully understood the instructions for each of the medications, especially how and when to take the medication. I could have interpreted the instructions simultaneously, but simultaneous interpreting by phone is very difficult because the nurse and I would be speaking at the same time, which would end up causing more confusion for the patient, if not for all of us. Thus, I ended up summarizing rather than interpreting word for word. Simultaneous interpreting works best only in person at the doctor's office or in court.

Case No. 3: Speak Slowly and Clearly Method (Consecutive Interpreting/Asking for Clarifications as Needed)

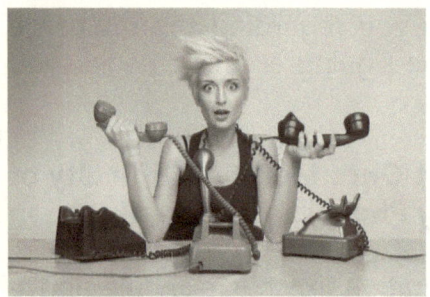

Patient: Zeej Tshoj Kim Kub (sixty-five-year-old male patient)

Nurse: Terry

Location: At the hospital with Dr. Doe

Interpreter: Niam Nkauj Zuag Paj

(At the hospital, the doctor appears to be an international doctor, as evident with his strong accent. There was also a static noise on the phone, which made it hard to hear the doctor clearly.)

(Phone ringing)

Interpreter: Hi, my name is Niam Nkauj Zuag Paj, and my ID number is 11211. When you are ready, please go ahead.

Nurse: Hi, my name is Terry, the nurse from the hospital who is taking care of Zeej Tshoj Kim Kub. He came to the hospital last night because he has heart and kidney failure. The doctor is coming right now. He is here now.

Doctor: Hi, my name is Dr. Doe.

Interpreter: Excuse me, Doctor, what is your name again?

Doctor: I am Dr. Doe.

Interpreter: Thank you, Doctor. *(After he repeated it, then I reinterpreted* exactly the *doctor said to the patient.)*

Doctor: I want the patient to know and understand that most of his organs inside are still okay, except his kidneys are completely gone. I want the patient to have dialysis now, or he will die.

Interpreter: Doctor, can you please repeated what you just said because I did not hear you very well. *(After he repeated it, then I reinterpreted* exactly the *doctor said to the patient.)*

Patient: I do not think that he knows what he is talking about. If what he just said was true, then I should be dead by now. But why I am still alive here today if both of my kidneys are completely dead like he said? If both my kidneys were completely gone, I would not be sitting right here right now. I am not a doctor, but I know that if one of the parts inside a person's body was dead, then that person is dead already. No,

I refuse to do the dialysis because I know many of my cousins and friends who had dialysis done, and they all had died. If I decide to do the dialysis, I know I will die just like the rest of the people that I know, so that is why I do not want to go through dialysis. I would rather want to die peacefully instead of letting the doctor cut and open me up first.

Interpreter: Doctor, I still have a very difficult time hearing from you. Please repeat everything again. (*After he repeated it, I then reinterpreted everything to the patient.*)

Doctor: Again, both his kidneys were already dead a month ago. I am trying to help him, so that is why I gave him the advice and suggestion to do the dialysis. But if he does not want it, he needs to go home and die at home.

Interpreter: Doctor, I am very sorry. I still cannot hear you that well. Please repeat what you just said again. (*After the doctor repeated, I reinterpreted everything that the doctor said to the patient.*)

Patient: Okay, I want to go home right now too. This doctor does not know what he is talking?

Interpreter: (Interpreted exactly what the patient said to the doctor.)

Analysis for Case No. 3: Speak Slow and Clear Method (Consecutive Interpreting/Asking for Clarifications as Needed)

This particular case was a great challenge for me. My job is to clearly communication between medical professionals and patients. However, I felt that my job was greatly compromised because not only did the phone have static, the doctor's accent was also very strong. When the doctor started speaking, I could not hear and understand what he was saying at all due to his thick accent. Furthermore, while he was talking, I just heard lots of static that sounded like rain in the background. This made it even more difficult to understand him at all. I felt bad that every time after he spoke, I had to ask him to please repeat what he had just said. If I did not ask him to repeat, I was completely in the dark and did not understand a single word from him well.

The main problem was the doctor's heavy accent, but I did not want to tell them that I had a problem understanding him. I would feel very embarrassed, and I might have made him feel embarrassed too. What I learned in this case was that, as an interpreter, I had to identify what was challenging my ability to understand the medical encounter. I worked hard to not embarrass or shame anyone. I kept on trying to understand the content of the information by asking the doctor to repeat himself, even though I did not feel good doing it. It would greatly help me if medical professionals who have thick accents speak slowly and clearly to ensure that the interpreter understands; or even asking if the interpreter understands what has been said. Maybe even start out by saying, I have an accent, so if you have a hard time understanding me, please ask me to repeat or speak slower. This would be most helpful. It would lighten up the encounter very much.

Case No. 4: Talk-to-the-Appropriate-Person Method (Know How and Whom to Ask for the Information You Seek)

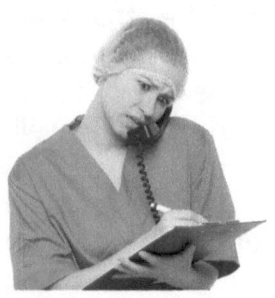

Patient: Tooj Kub Hlau (seventy-two-year-old male patient who will have a surgery)

Interpreter: Niam Nkauj Zuag Paj

Nurse: Marthatia

(Phone ringing)

Interpreter: Hi, my name is Niam Nkauj Zuag Paj, and my ID number is 11211. When you are ready, please go ahead.

Nurse: My name is Marthatia, and I am a nurse at the hospital. I need to call this patient to talk to him regarding his surgery tomorrow. His name is Tooj Kub Hlau. His phone is 999-999-9999.

Interpreter: Okay, can you please hold for a minute while I dial the patient's phone number?

Nurse: Yes.

(Phone ringing)

Patient: Hello.

Interpreter: Hi, I am a Hmong interpreter lady, and there is also a nurse from the hospital with me on the phone right now. Is Tooj Kub Hlau available?

Patient: This is Tooj Kub Hlau.

Interpreter: Tooj Kub Hlau, the reason why we are calling you today is regarding your surgery tomorrow. Is this a good time for us to talk to you regarding your appointment now?

Patient: Yes.

Interpreter: Nurse, I am talking to the patient now, please go right ahead with your questions.

Nurse: Hi, Tooj Kub Hlau. My name is Marthatia. I am calling from your surgeon's office where you are coming to have your surgery tomorrow. I would like to know if you already have your pre-op exam done with your primary physician yet. If you did already, where did you get it done? What is the name of the clinic? Who is the doctor? Do you remember the doctor's name? Do you have the clinic's phone number?

Interpreter: (Interpreted exactly to the patient what the nurse said.)

Patient: Yes, I did have the pre-op exam done last week already. The clinic was over there. It was located behind the two big trees next to Wal-Mart and Dollar Tree Store. When you drive on the freeway you can see the clinic over there. I did not know the name of the clinic and the doctor's name because I did not know how to read or write. Every time I made the appointment and went to see my doctor, they always changed new doctors, so I did not know my doctor's name. There are too many doctors working there, so I do not know who my doctor is. The nurse should have all of the information since she knows how to read and write. Why does she still ask me all of these questions? If she wants to know, she can come and take me there. I can show where the place is to her. If I know how to read and write like her, I would never ask these questions.

Interpreter: (Interpreted exactly what the patient said to the nurse.)

Nurse: Do you know the time and the place that you are coming to have your surgery tomorrow at? Your appointment is 9:00 a.m., but we would like you to be there at 7:30 a.m. in the morning. Have you ever had any high fever in your family history? Do you have any allergy like seasonal or food problems? Are you having any asthma now? Are you taking any medications? If you are taking medications, why you are taking them? How have you been taking them? What are the names of your medications? Are you using any alcoholics, drugs, or marijuana? Do you ever smoke? In your family history, do any of your family members or you have these health problems as following: strokes, stomachache, kidneys, heart, diabetes, blood pressure, brain damage, anxiety, depression, sexual transmit, blood disorder, Hepatitis A, B, or C?

Interpreter: (Interpreted exactly what the nurse said to the patient.)

Patient: Why does this nurse ask too many questions? I do not know if I have these health problems or not because when we used to live in Laos, we did not have doctors; so we never went to see a doctor for our illnesses to see what diseases we had. If I have these problems, I would let her know, but I do not know. Now that I am in America, I always go to see my doctor at his office when I am sick, so she should have all my information from his office by now. If she still wants any other information, why does she call my doctor's office? Regarding my medications, I am taking a lot of different kinds of pills right now. I do not know how to read, so I do not know the name of the medications. My children are the ones who give them for me to take only. They are at work now, so if the nurse wants to know the names of my medications, she can call back when they are coming from work. My son will come home from work at 11:00 p.m., and my daughter-in-law will come home from work at 8:30 p.m. The nurse should know that I do not speak English, and so she should call when my children are home. I want to know why she keeps asking me too many of these questions. If she continues asking me these questions, I will probably have heart attack right now because I am very worried about my surgery tomorrow and already have tons of pressures for myself now, so I cannot think about anything else at this moment at all. Like I said, I cannot read and write, so I cannot take any notes from her or give her any information that she needs from me. Since I do not know how to read and write, I do not know exactly what information she wants from me. Why does she call so late in the day? She should call early this morning while my children are still here. Tell the nurse that I am a Vietnam veteran. I used to help the Americans during the Vietnam War, so Americans should help and save me. Does she know that I and many other Hmong soldiers saved so many American soldiers in the jungle when their planes crashed and they got injured? I almost died in the war, but the reason I did not die was because I was a very honest person by helping the American soldiers, and my ancestors saved me. Please tell the nurse to help me through this surgery because I do not want to die yet.

Interpreter: (Interpreted exactly what the patient said to the nurse.)

Nurse: Does he know how tall he is and how much he weighs? Does he have health insurance? If he comes tomorrow, please wear loose clothes and leave all valuable items at home. He must have a family member or a friend to come with him and stay home with him in the first twenty-four hours after the surgery. He cannot eat or drink anything by midnight tonight. Please bring all of his medication bottles with him tomorrow morning so his doctor will know exactly what medications he is taking. Again, does he know the surgery place tomorrow, right?

Interpreter: (Interpreted exactly what the nurse said to the patient.)

Patient: Interpreter, can you explain to her that she asks too many questions from me and I cannot give them to her because I do not know. I already told her that I do not speak any words of English so I do not know how much I weight or how tall I am. My children know everything and have all of my information, so they will bring whatever I have with me for the surgery tomorrow. Can she stop asking me any more questions? Otherwise, I will hang up on her if she keeps asking too many questions.

Interpreter: (Interpreted exactly what the patient said to the nurse.)

Nurse: Ok.

Analysis for Case No. 4: Talk-to-the-Appropriate-Person Method (Know How and Whom to Ask for the Information You Seek)

This elderly Hmong male patient did not speak English at all and did not understand how the Western cultures in the medical field works. When the nurse called and wanted to verify so much information from him before he went to his surgery appointment, he did not understand. As a result, he got very upset and felt very frustrated as to why the nurse kept asking so many questions. One of the main reasons that the patient got very upset and very frustrated was because he did not know how to speak, read, and write in English; and he did not know where to find the information for her because it was his children that managed his medications.

For example, he did not even know the name of the medications that he was taking, but the nurse kept asking him to spell the names of the medications to her over the phone. From the nurse's point of view, it was also very frustrating for her too because in order for the patient to have the surgery done tomorrow, he had to provide the information to her before he could have the surgery. The main reasons were that the nurse wanted to know and make sure he did not have any major or serious sickness at the present time. The nurse also needed to account for the names of the medications that he is taking right before the surgery, reminded him to bring all important information to his appointment, explained the surgery procedure before and after to him, and provided the location of his surgery to him.

As an interpreter, I understood both parties' frustrations very well. As the middle person who helps to bridge the medical gap, I would like to suggest to both parties that, first, the nurse needed to take more time to explain slowly to the patient how the surgery procedure works from start to end in order to make sure the patient understands her points clearly. Second, the nurse should explain why it is important to ask so many questions to the patient about his health history. And third, the nurse should have listened to the patient telling her that it is his children who managed his care and that she should call them to obtain the information she was seeking.

Chapter Three

Closing Thoughts on the Challenges of Interpreting Different Worldviews

I am very glad that my role as the interpreter is meant to ease and facilitate the communication between the limited or non–English-speaking Hmong patient and American medical staffs. If it were not for people like me who can speak two languages, communication would be extremely difficult for people who only spoke one language but live in a multilingual society. It is with this purpose in mind that sharing my experiences as a Hmong interpreter is so important to me. If I don't share my experiences about the challenges and rewards of being a Hmong interpreter, how can we (interpreter and/or translator, medical staff, hospitals, et al) meet the needs of patients? It is only through examining what is working and what is not working within the system that we can learn from it and/or strengthen it.

I have learned that interpreting is not only the process of carrying the message and meaning from one language into another; but it is also the interpretation of one cultural context into another. Therefore, interpreters have a dual job of correct interpretation, and also cultural education, assistance and facilitation. This job gets compounded by the different cultural worldviews that the interpreter has to navigate, and make on-the-spot decisions about what is crucial to attend to and what is not. This requires a high level of bi-cultural competency.

In the United States of America, when Americans get sick, they seek out medical doctors to find out exactly what illness they have. When American patients get sick, they call to make an appointment, and then go to see their primary physician. Upon arrival, we would park our cars in the lot, walk into our doctor's office and go straight to the receptionist's window. We would give our insurance card to the receptionist to verify all our personal information, and then wait patiently until one of the medical assistants calls for us to go in to one of the exam rooms in the back. While we go into the exam room, we keep waiting until the doctor comes in. The moment the doctor comes into the room to talk to us patients, the doctor would say, "What is wrong today?" We, the patients, would say that we either have a headache or have had a cough for a week. The doctor would take a look at our throats and ears, and listen to our heart and lungs. It is a common practice that during doctor visits, we will discuss our health problems, including symptoms and onset of illness. Most of the time, medical doctors are able to help us get well by prescribing medication to get rid of the illness. Sometimes when doctors cannot see what is making us sick, they have to go inside our bodies through the use of special devices or take x-rays to see the inside of our bodies to find out what exactly is causing us to be sick.

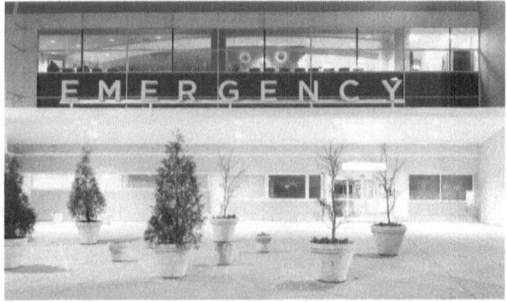

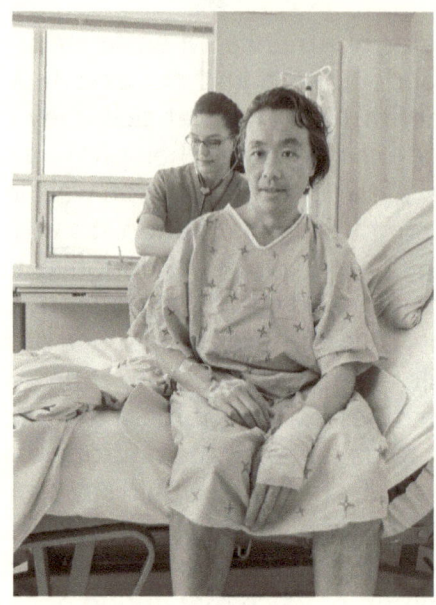

As Hmong people have adapted to the new culture in America, we have also come to understand and use this Western medical model. However, for our older Hmong patients who have lived most of their lives in Laos, they still believe that natural remedies are the best medicine for health-care problems. In every clan, there is usually an elder that is the medicine man or woman who has great knowledge about all sorts of natural remedies; elders know and practice using herbs and plants to heal the body. Elders often boil these natural herbs and plants in a cooking pot for a very long time, after which we then drink the liquid to improve or cure the disease inside our body. Elders also blanch these special natural herbs and plants and wrap it around the part of the body that is in pain to heal the skin and muscles. For the older Hmong generation, because their perspective on healing is different, going to the doctor's office is the last resort—which means that when they do go, their health condition may have become poor, and they may not always follow through with the medication instructions.

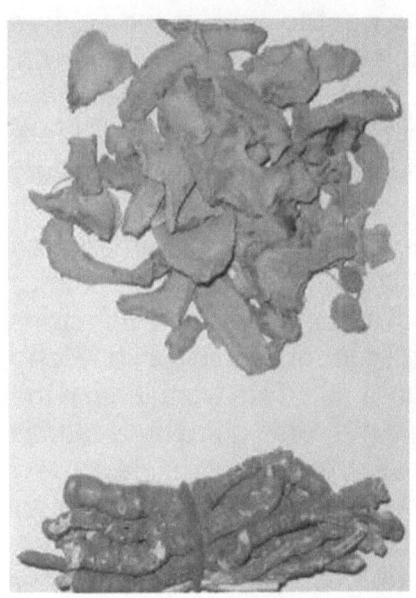
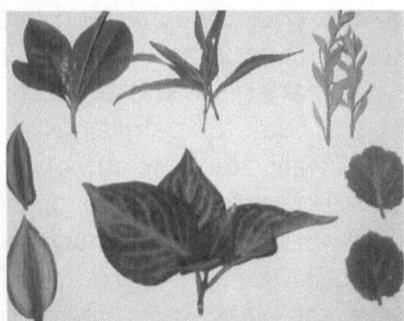

"Author's Own Photos": Sample pictures of barks and plants that the Hmong people use for medicinal purposes.

Furthermore, the communication style of Hmong people is very circular and indirect, which oftentimes conflict with the American style of communication, which is often very direct. Hmong elders like to share their whole life story from their childhood until now because they want to make sure that their doctors fully understand them and the origin of their illness. For example, the patient begins to tell her story about how she got her back pains to the nurse. She begins by telling her life story that as a little girl she had to go work very hard at the field, carried too much heavy stuff on her back, and sometimes babysat for her siblings while her parents went to work in the fields. When the doctor finally comes in to the examination room, he begins to ask the patient a lot of questions: "Did you fall?" "How did you get these back pains?" "How long ago did you have this pain?" The patient answers, "I remember when I was about six or seven years old then, I used to carry a basket full of rice, corns, and other vegetables from the field. Sometimes I also carried my siblings at home while my parents went to work at the field. At home, early in the morning and right before the sun went down, I took an empty bucket to go to the stream to carry water to my house to cook breakfast and dinner for my family. After all those duties in Laos, I arrived in Thailand and came to America; every day, my back pains started hurting me more and more than ever before. Today, the pain is never gone for a second. Sometimes I cannot walk, stand up straight, and sit for too long. Sometimes if I lie down on the sofa or bed for a while, then the pains would not hurt me that much, but I cannot lie down all day long because I have things to do too. Right now, I am wondering if the doctor can please help me and give me some good medications for my back pains." Despite the patient trying to provide context for the pain, fifteen minutes in to the conversation, the doctor is ready to leave the exam room. As he is heading to the door, he says that he is going to prescribe two prescriptions for her back pains. The first medication is Tylenol with codeine, and the second one is to relax her muscles.

It is difficult to pinpoint the exact issues: Is it the different communication styles? Is it the limited time, which doctors have available to spend with patients? Is it the different worldviews about health and healing? In reality, it is probably a combination of all of these factors that contribute to a challenging healthcare situation. Perhaps over time, these interpreting and cultural differences will be less of an issue due to patient acculturation. In the meantime, the intersection of these issues cannot be ignored. We must consciously attend to the various cultural differences and examine how these different views and ways of communicating can either hinder or support patient care. Together, we must come up with solutions that will aid all sides—medical providers, interpreters, and patients—in working effectively together. It is my hope that by sharing my personal experiences as a Hmong interpreter in the medical field and other areas, this will help provide some helpful insights and assistance or solutions to the various language and cultural complexities and difficulties.

Epilogue

I decided to write this book because as an over-the-phone interpreter who processes and facilitates language meanings and critical information between our Hmong culture and our Western culture, I have realized that there can be so many misunderstandings during the interpretation sessions. Because we do not communicate in the same language, may not think the same way, or may not be seeing the world through the same eyes. Interestingly, when I used to interpret face-to-face in the past for our Hmong patients, it was not as hard as over-the-phone. In person, I could use my facial expressions, hand gestures, and body language to communicate in order to get the message across between the two different languages and cultures.

As an over-the-phone interpreter, I feel like I am a blind person because I cannot see the faces of the doctors, nurses, or other professional staffs and the older non–English-speaking Hmong patients. The moment the phone rings and I answer the call, I must listen carefully to the caller's situation, and I must use my imagination quickly to access the situation in order for me to interpret correctly. Sometimes when the weather is bad or there is static over the phone, my job becomes more challenging because it is very difficult to hear the callers' voices clearly. When the bad weather and static are combined with people who view the world very differently from each other, then I have a major problem on hand.

When I interpret for two different languages and cultures, the biggest problem for me is when the older non–English-speaking Hmong patients and medical staffs do not see things in a similar manner. It is like comparing apples to oranges. Let us put it in this way for clarification. For the older Hmong patients, they think the world is flat because they go by how they are living on this Earth, where they are standing under their own two feet on the ground, and how they see the Earth. On the other hand, for the American medical staffs, they think and know that the world is round because they have done tons of researches and understand how complex and different the world is. In fact, all of the older non–English-speaking Hmong knowledge shows them that the Earth is round. For them, they go by what they can see and feel; but the medical staffs go by what the data, as evidences, prove to them.

When the older and uneducated Hmong patients and the medical staffs have to interact, not only do they speak totally different languages, their two worldviews are also so different. So although the medical staffs might just want me to interpret verbatim, I end up having to also interpret culturally. Only by doing this can we make sure everyone is on the same page. It is great that medical professionals respect patients' rights and want to make sure they fully understand their medical conditions or situations, but many of them are not aware of or sensitive to the cultural differences in worldview.

While I know that during the interpreting process, each of us has a role in either making the process easier or more challenging, I hope that this book will offer some helpful and useful insights and solutions for the medical professionals, because they have the responsibility of patient care in terms of how to best utilize the professional language interpreter, their education and professional trainings to understand the cultural perspective of older non–English-speaking Hmong patients. It is through this process of critical analysis of the interpreting process and conscious awareness that they can then more effectively achieve their medical mission of great patient care.

I also would like to encourage our younger Hmong generation today, who sometimes end up interpreting or translating for older family members, to remember to not only interpret or translate correctly so as not to lose the critical message or meaning, but also to ensure that the underlying cultural messages get across and are understood. It is also important to explain to our older Hmong patients how everything works in the medical field, so hopefully, when our older Hmong patients see their primary physicians or ER doctors, they will focus and be more direct about their current illnesses rather than tell their whole life story. Lastly, I would like the medical field to recognize the fact that sometimes language interpretation cannot be verbatim and that a little extra time is needed to ensure cultural understanding.

My average incoming calls-per-day is probably about fifteen to twenty calls. As a Hmong interpreter, I do not mind how many calls are coming each day; the most important thing for me is to be able to help both parties. I am an older Hmong woman who understands very well how difficult it is for our grandparents and parents, who do not speak much English, to get good and critical medical care. I am very glad to be the middle person who passes the critical messages or meanings between both parties—medical providers and non–English-speaking Hmong patients. I believe it is my job to not only interpret verbatim, but also to provide the very best cultural explanation and assistance whenever it is needed. I also strongly believe that it is my responsibility to also share with others the lessons that I have learned. I do believe that it is only when all of us do our part and share our learned knowledge that true understanding can be achieved, and then the best care possible will be available for the non–English-speaking patients and at the same time provide rewarding experiences for the providers and interpreter or translator alike.

www.ingramcontent.com/pod-product-compliance
Lightning Source LLC
Chambersburg PA
CBHW030911180526
45163CB00004B/1784